COMPLETE GUIDE
to healthy
HAIR

"There is so much more to beautiful hair than genetics and luck! In fact, our hair is a window into our 'inner' health, physical and emotional, providing clues as to the road ahead. This book provides a clear path to follow to achieve luxuriant locks along with some surprising and life-transforming insights."

SALLY GRAY ND, DUNSBOROUGH, WESTERN-AUSTRALIA, NATUROPATH, NUTRITIONIST AND TRANSPERSONAL COUNSELOR

"Do you also believe that everything is possible? Did someone once tell you that your hair is too thin? Did you get recommended not to let it grow longer again? Then this is your book to read, and learn how beautiful your hair is! Lies Helsloot is living proof that you can always achieve what you wish for."

SASKIA WINKLER, GERMANY, COACH AND MENTOR

FOR FURTHER INFORMATION

WWW.TAKEYOUTIME.COM

Sally Gray ND: **WWW.SALLYGRAYND.COM**

Saskia Winkler, coach and mentor: **WWW.SASKIA-WINKLER.COM**

Haylie Pomroy, nutritionist: **WWW.HAYLIEPOMROY.COM**

Jack Canfield, life coach and author: **WWW.JACKCANFIELD.COM**

The COMPLETE GUIDE to healthy HAIR

A 3-STEP PROGRAM TO HEAL YOUR HAIR

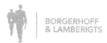 BORGERHOFF & LAMBERIGTS

LIES HELSLOOT

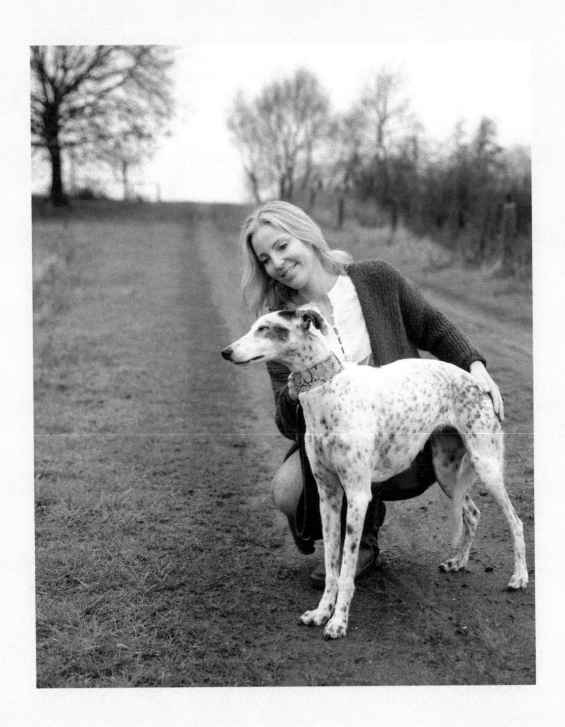

INTRO 7

LET'S TALK ABOUT HAIR 15

WHAT IS A HAIR? FROM GROWTH TO DECAY... 16

BLACK, RED OR BLONDE?
HOW IS THE COLOR OF YOUR HAIR MADE? 23

HAIR STRUCTURE: STRAIGHT, WAVY OR FRIZZY 24

FOOD FOR HAIR 43

THE IMPORTANCE OF HEALTHY AND BALANCED NUTRITION 46

EAT! 51

WATER: THE HEALTHY THIRST QUENCHER AND SOURCE OF LIFE 77

HERBS AND HERBAL MEDICINE FOR YOUR HAIR 80

HAIRCARE 89

TAKE YOU TIME 131

OUR BUSY LIFE 134

TAPPING OR EFT (Emotional Freedom Technique) 140

EXERCISES 162

RECIPES FOR HEALTHY HAIR 171

COCONUT-ALOE HAIR MASK 175

AVOCADO-EGG-HONEY MASK 177

MORE VOLUME: THE BELGIAN WAY 179

CHAMOMILE MASK FOR NATURAL HIGHLIGHTS 181

NETTLE WATER 183

MAMA-MIX: RECIPE OF MY SPECIAL HERBAL TEA 185

DIVINE OIL-TREATMENT AND MORE... 186

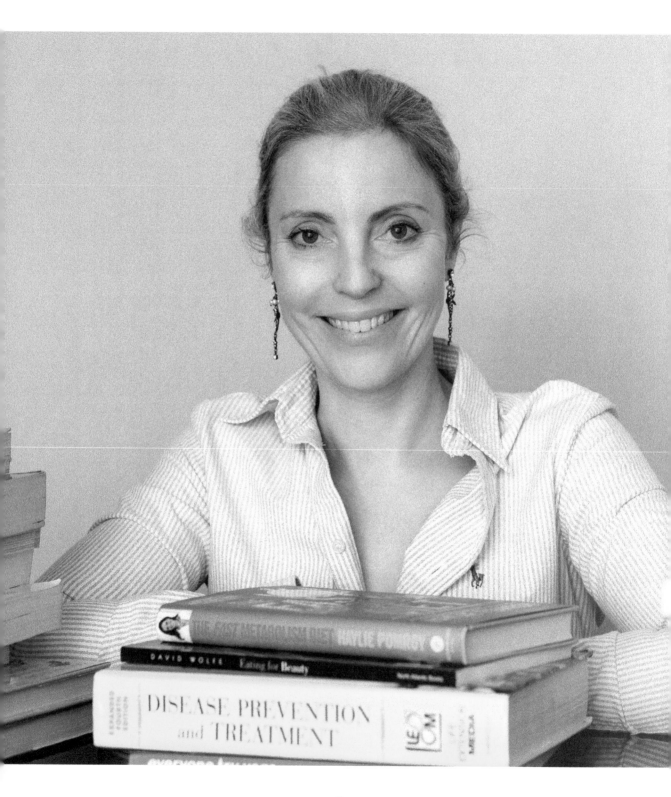

INTRO

I am crazy about hair! When I was a young girl, I was called 'the girl with the long hair', because in my younger years (although I don't feel old at all now!) I indeed had extremely long and shiny hair. Everyone always asked me about my secret. Throughout the years, with some extra birthdays on my calendar and especially after the birth of my beautiful daughter, my hair started to change.

It was thinning, very brittle and dry, I could fill pillows with the hair I lost every day and my scalp was super-sensitive. It was driving me mad. That is exactly the moment where my quest began, my quest for the secret of healthy, shiny and strong hair. This journey brought me back to 'the roots'.

When I look back on my life track, it wasn't exactly linear. I studied Political and Social Sciences at the University of Ghent, but I always had a real passion for the beauty of nature, health, nutrition, exercise and spirituality. In 2003 I did an acquisition of a healthy restaurant, Avalon, in the heart of the historic center of the city of Ghent and became proficient in the power of tasty, healthy food. I saw the positive health effect of my cuisine on my clients and this made me intensely happy and satisfied. It was my contribution to a better, healthier world.

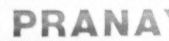

After I sold the business at the end of 2008 to its current owners, a couple of passionate health foodies and food lovers, I started to indulge in the topic of health. The link between health and a healthy head of hair was one of the things I wanted to research more in-depth.

I wanted to know everything there was to know about hair and for a couple of years I studied everything I could find on the topic. I took courses in ortho-molecular medicine and refined my knowledge in healthy food I had acquired in my previous career in my healthy restaurant and as a private health chef. I also started a spiritual journey to myself because I noticed that the stress of my daily life as a single mom in a challenging 'living together apart family', as an entrepreneur and a busy bee was taking its toll on my body. My body and mind were completely exhausted and I had reached the limits of my strength. My body was out of balance: pregnancy, the birth process, breastfeeding and taking care of a child certainly had their role in this.

To make things even worse, a couple of maltreatments and poor colorings totally ruined my hair. It made me very curious about the reasons behind it.

I studied, played guinea pig and experienced myself what issues had the greatest impact on my hair. All these findings I share with you because I think you can benefit from my tips. There must be a reason why you picked this book from the shelve.

During these times I also rediscovered one of my older secrets: daily brushing with a quality hairbrush. Because I couldn't find one that met my criteria, another project sprouted out of my search and it will become reality around the same time this book goes to press: my own line of hairbrushes, made in Belgium, top quality, called Delphin & Emerence. A nice proof that things in life happen as they are meant to be and especially a confirmation of one of my life mantras: 'one thing leads to another' and 'sometimes you just have to hold your nose and jump'.

In short, I went on a search for 'the how' and 'the why' and 'the better'. All my experiences can be read in this beautiful book. The book is about my story, my quest. I am not a doctor, nor a dermatologist or a trichologist (=hair expert), but thanks to the support of a couple of experts behind the screens, I was able to fill this book with tried and tested methods. Therefore I am convinced that all of my experiences and tips will help you get or maintain a healthy head of hair. I wrote this book for all the busy, ambitious, interesting, cool and especially fantastic women who are looking for balance in their lives. It deeply touches me when I hear women say that there is nothing they can do about the fact that their hair is thinning and going brittle and that it is a part of the ageing process that has to be accepted. I want to show you that there is another way. So… let it shine!

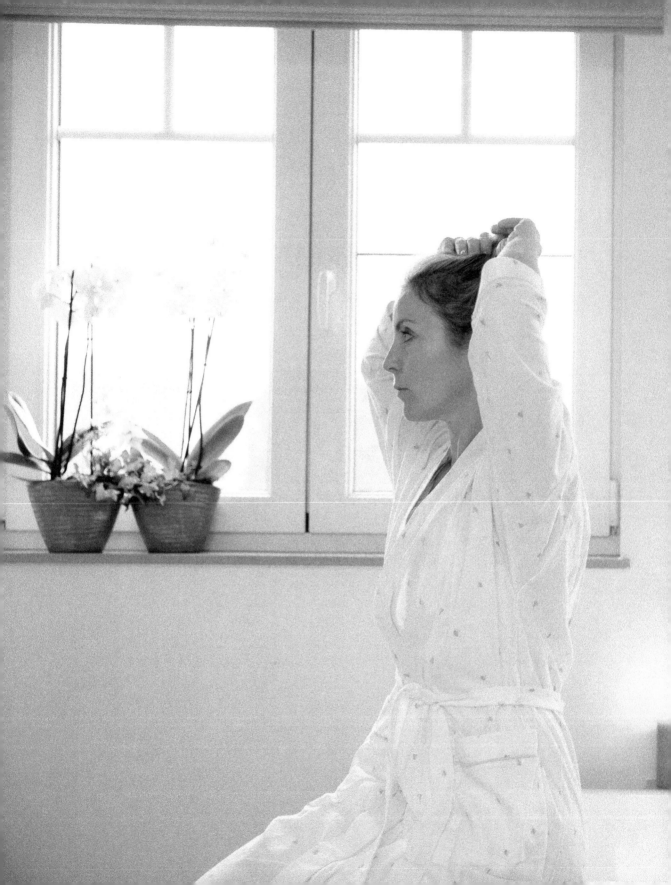

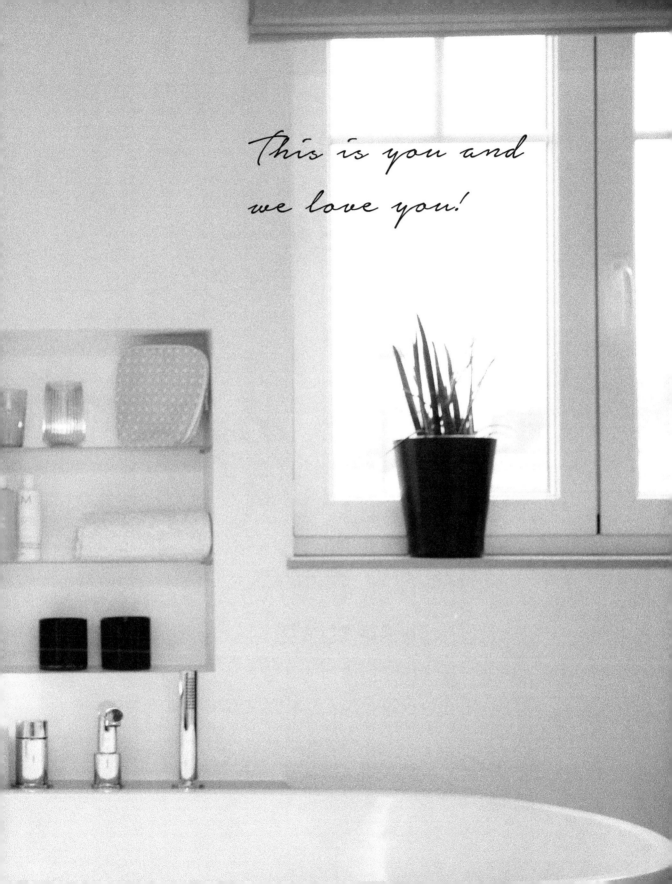

This is you and
we love you!

Invest in

it is the

never take

your hair,

crown you

off.

LET'S
TALK
ABOUT
HAIR

WHAT IS A HAIR?
FROM GROWTH TO DECAY...

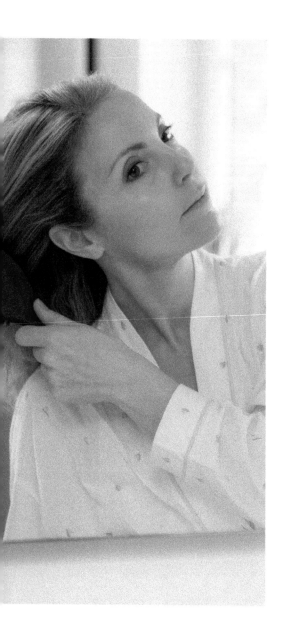

I will start this book with a bit of basic knowledge about head hair before I unveil my three-step program. I think it is very important that you have at least some knowledge of how a hair is built, how the growth process works and what can go wrong during this process. Knowing this was important in my own search to the 'how' and 'why' of my own hair issues. It will help you in the next chapters to understand why certain things have an influence on the condition of your hair. If you want to know more 'hair tips', you can always follow my blog at www.takeyoutime.com.

The scientific study of hair is called 'trichology'. This branch of science studies the hair in all its different aspects and takes a closer look at the hair itself, at the scalp and at the different metabolic processes that go with it. A hair is more than the part you can see with the human eye. A hair starts to grow from the hair follicle. The follicle is the only 'living' part of the hair, because the hair shaft itself, the visible part of the hair, is actually dead material. The structure in and around the follicle is a complex thing.

The follicle is surrounded by tiny blood vessels that supply it with oxygen and nutrients. Around the follicle, tiny little muscles make sure you get goosebumps (from that handsome actor or gorgeous actress) on your legs and arms and make the hair of your head 'stand up' when you get startled. It is also those muscles that make sure the sebaceous glands around the hair base excrete 'sebum', your own natural and

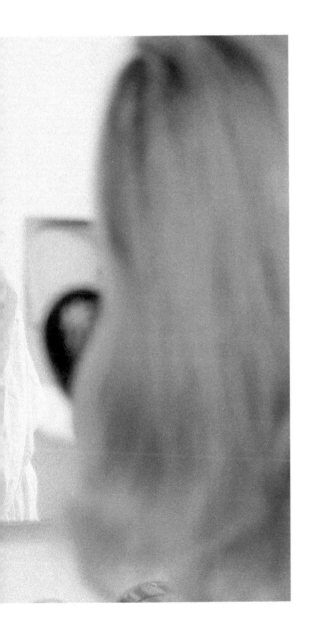

self-made caring oil, rich in nutrients like essential fatty acids, natural waxes and vitamin E to nourish your hair and make sure the hair cuticles are lying flat, making your hair shine. Sebum is also a naturally waterproof product that makes your hair less frizzy. It also transports vitamin E to your hair and skin. Vitamin E is a very important vitamin to combat the skin ageing process. As a result, it is a common ingredient in cosmetic products.

Exactly there, in that follicle and especially in its base called the 'papilla', the cycle of hair growth will start and exists of four phases, which we will discuss later on:

- the **anagen phase**

- the **catagen phase**

- the **telogen phase**

- the **exogen phase.**

The hair itself is built from a protein, which is named 'keratin'. This protein is known for the easy absorption of liquids. This is why your hair structure looks different and longer when your hair is wet. Your hair will take its original structure when it's dry again. At the base of the hair, you have the root that connects the hair to the follicle.

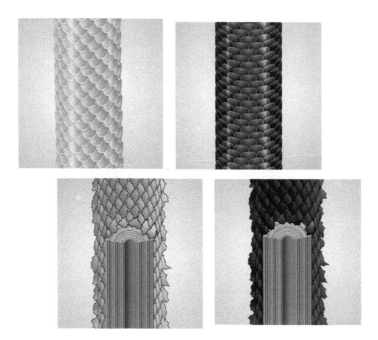

The innermost layer of the hair is named the 'medulla' (hair marrow) and around that is the 'cortex' or 'hair bark'. The cortex consists of a series of long-stretched cells that, when combined, form into strands. These strands of cells are called, macro- and microfibers. These fibers are connected to each other through a sort of cement-like substance (matrix). All the way on the outside are the hair sheaths. You can compare these sheaths to roofing tiles. These sheaths form an important protection layer around the medulla and the cortex to protect them against external influences. The sheaths are a natural way to keep moisture in the hair.

The number of hair sheaths differs per hair type. People with Asian hair have the most hair sheaths, up next are the Afro hair textures and all the way at the bottom of the list are the Caucasian types. These differences have an impact on how hair behaves under different circumstances and tell us how you can provide the best care for this type of hair.

When the hair sheaths are lying flat, your hair will look much better than when the hair sheaths are 'straight up'. The hair sheaths must be open to color your hair and to make hair color penetrate deep into the hair. Certain hair volume treatments give the same effect. The hair sheaths need to close after such a treatment, which is important to achieve a smooth and shiny result. Later on more about that.

Just like the human skin consists of a vast array of different colors and textures, there are many differences in hair structure. The frizzy hair of African, Afro-American and North-African types is clearly different from the fine, blonde hair from the far north. Asians mostly have smooth and thick hair. Every hair type has different needs, because of the different structure. An adjusted treatment for styles, colors, caretaking and brushing.

Let us have a closer look at the different phases, which I mentioned earlier on.

THE ANAGEN PHASE

This is the phase in which the 'papilla' builds a new hair shaft and the hair starts to grow until it reaches a genetically determined length. Depending on where the hair grows on your body, it will reach a certain length. Your eyebrow has a shorter maximum length than the hair on your head. In this book we will only talk about the hair on your head. Head hair grows the fastest of all body hair and can grow the longest. It can grow up to 80 centimeters (31.5 inches) in women. It will grow a bit shorter in men, until a maximum length of 50 centimeters (19.70 inches). There are exceptions where the hair grows even longer. Everyone has a genetically determined maximum length. This is the reason why some people can grow their hair longer than others. According to the *Guinness Book of Records* the Chinese Xie Quiping owns the record for the longest hair, which measures 5.627 meters (18 feet, 5.54 inches). She has been growing her hair from the age of 13, then 1973. These circumstances are highly exceptional, but they do occur.

When I was a young girl, I could grow my hair very long without any trouble, but some of my girlfriends would never reach this length.

A head hair will grow an average of 0.35 millimeters (0.014 inches) a day or, depending on the hair type, up to 1 to 1.4 centimeters (0.40 to 0.55 inches) per month. The hair growth of most people will be between 12 to 15 centimeters (4.7 to 6 inches) per year, depending on age and health. The younger you are, the quicker it will grow. The length of the anagen growth phase is different for each person and can go from two to six years.

The hair of the Asian type grows the fastest (1.4 cm/0.55 inches per month on average), followed by the Caucasian hair type (1.2 cm/0.47 inches on average per month) and lastly the African type of hair (with an average of 0.9 cm/0.35 inches per month).

A head has an average of 80,000 to 150,000 hairs. The number of hairs per person is connected to the color of your hair. As a result, people with ginger-colored hair have less hair (between 80,000 and 90,000) and blondes have the most (140,000 on average). Luckily, Mother Nature made sure that not all the hairs are in the same phase, this explains that some hairs are fully growing and some are in one of the next phases.

At the moment that a hair reaches its maximum length, the growth phase will stop and the hair will reach the catagen phase.

THE CATAGEN PHASE

In the catagen phase the hair papilla will stop producing hair shaft cells and the bottom region of the hair papilla will start to shrink in an upward motion to the surface of the scalp. The catagen phase is a short one, which will take only several days. At that moment the papilla will enter a resting phase.

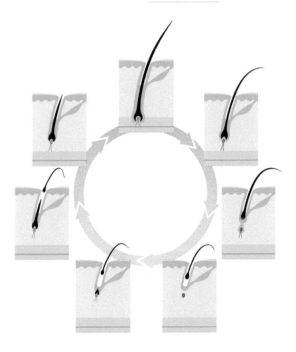

THE TELOGEN PHASE

At the moment the catagen phase ends, the papilla will enter a rest phase where no more cell growth or cell division will occur. The hair will stop growing. This phase can take weeks up to months. On average, about 10 to 15% of the hair papilla are in rest.

THE LAST PHASE: THE EXOGEN PHASE

This phase is mostly seen as a part of the telogen phase, but I will discuss this separately. Because the papilla enters a new growth phase, a hair will start to grow underneath the 'old' hair in the resting phase. Due to the growth of the new hair, the hair shaft will detach itself from the papilla and make the hair fall out. That's when the cycle starts all over again.

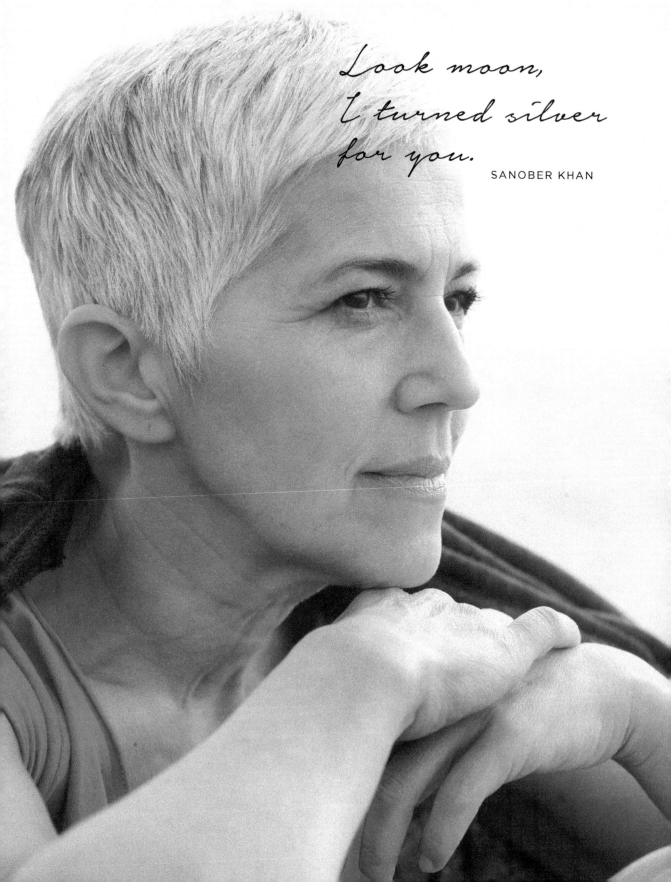

Look moon,
I turned silver
for you.

SANOBER KHAN

BLACK, RED OR BLONDE?? HOW IS THE COLOR OF YOUR HAIR MADE??

The hair cortex contains a substance called 'melanin', which determines the color of your hair. At the bottom of the hair root, pigments are being produced by pigmentation cells.

When your hair grows, your hair color will appear. You have two different kinds of melanin: 'eumelanin' and 'phaeomelanin'. They're located between the fibres in the cortex. Dark-haired people received more eumelanin while blondes and redheads, received more phaeomelanin.

HELP! They have arrived: white and grey hairs

Due to the ageing process, the production of pigments will stop. That is how your hair becomes grey or white. While one person will look very sexy with grey or white locks, the other person has a less fresh appearance. Grey hairs usually come later in life, but I got mine in my early thirties. Because I have blonde highlights, it's less noticeable. In the beginning I did color my hair, but over time I have decided to make them a part of me. It's up to you to decide if you choose to color your hair or let your new natural color grow out.

Your hairdresser is the best person to give you advice on how to support this process in a positive way and to enhance your new color with that little bit of 'oomph', which will make you shine. Have a look at inspiring examples like Helen Mirren, Diane Keaton, Jamie Lee Curtis, Christine Lagarde and Meryl Streep and the way in which they make grey and white hair part of their sparkling personality. Maybe it is time for some new outfits and an adjusted make-up that can bring your new look to life? You might also consider visiting an image consultant or color specialist to help you with that.

HAIR STRUCTURE: STRAIGHT, WAVY OR FRIZZY

The beautiful diversity of people on this planet gives a whole array of hair textures with many differences in density, structure and growth rhythm. The shape of the cortex and the shape of your hair is being determined by the shape of the follicle. That is the reason why hair is either straight or rather curly. I will discuss the different types shortly. People with straight hair have round-shaped hair. The oval and other shaped hairs are generally more found with wavy and curly hair types.

AFRO HAIR

Classic Afro hair/African-American hair has a lower density than my own blonde hair for example. On average there are about 120-140 hairs per square centimeter (or 0.16 square inch). On average these types have about 60,000 follicles. Surprisingly, due to the dark skin tone and frizzy hair texture, you get the impression that these types have the most hair.

Afro hair grows slower than Asian and Caucasian hair. Because of the strong curly texture, the Afro hair looks shorter, while it is much longer when stretched. This type of hair doesn't grow very long. The maximum length is 30 centimeters (11.8 inches) at best. The hair implant is different and the hairs are very closely implanted next to each other, which makes them very difficult to brush. The shape of the hair, when cut in half, is most likely flat and oval to the shape of an ellipse. This is the main reason why it frizzes and curls.

That is why the hair knots easily and especially when it isn't well cared for, because then the hair sheaths are 'open', which makes the hair strands 'hook' together and tangle up.

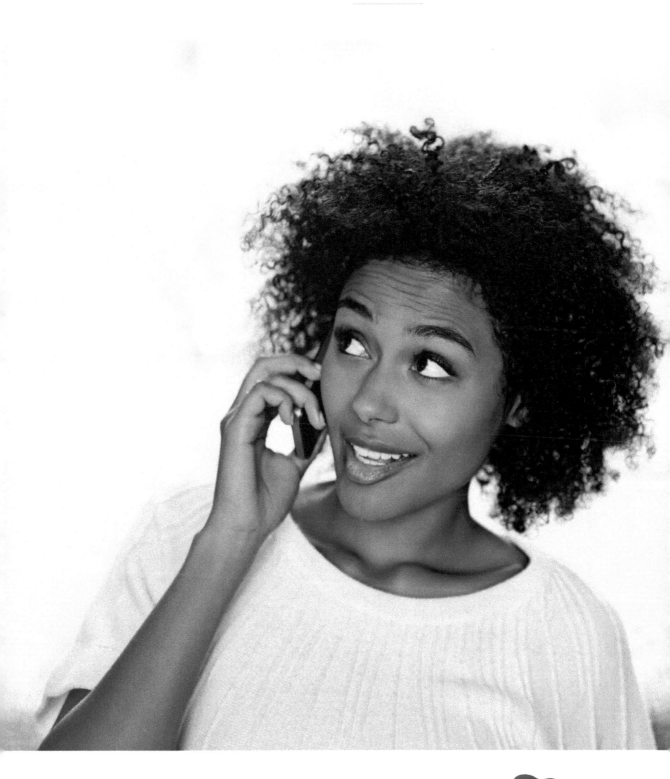

It is the most fragile hair type and is very prone to breakage, often due to harsh treatments and braiding. Whoever is blessed with beautiful Afro hair or North-African hair, has the most difficulty to spread sebum over the entire length of the hair through brushing. This is why a suitable hairbrush and good care of dry ends are very important for this type of hair.

ASIAN HAIR

This type of hair has an almost perfectly round shape. It is a type of hair that is mostly to be seen in Asia, but you can find it also in South American people and the native inhabitants of North America, the Indians. It is beautifully shiny, exceptionally strong and sleek hair, something blondes can only dream of. It is also the fastest growing hair type. The hair strands of these types are almost vertically implanted in the scalp. This makes it easy for short haircuts to 'stand up'. Asian hair is also blessed to grow the longest of all hair types. They have an average of 140 to 160 hairs per *square centimeter* (0.16 square inch) and a total of 80,000 follicles.

CAUCASIAN HAIR

Caucasian hair types have more follicles and thus more hair. Different sources give numbers from 200 up to an average of 227 hair strands per square centimeter (0.16 square inch). There are an average of 100,000 hair follicles on the scalp. This hair type can be identified by an oval shape of the hair shaft and the hair strands are implanted in a slanted way, which makes this type of hair the easiest to brush and spread sebum over the hair strands.

WHAT ABOUT OTHER TYPES?

There are so many different types of hair mixes, structures and colors that it is hard to give everyone a label. I'm not a fan of labelling everything myself. Each category has many differences, but no stress, because there is perfect care for each type of hair.

Embrace your true nature

We are all unique and were given our own special hair structure by Mother Nature. But so very often we aren't very satisfied with what we received. If you have straight hair, you want curls, if you have curls you want straight hair. If you are blessed with beautiful dark, frizzy hair you want to look like that blonde actress with straight hair... In short, we compare ourselves with role models who don't match our own natural beauty.

Going against nature isn't helpful for the quality of your hair and it kills your self-esteem. I notice this destructive behaviour in women who will do anything to look like model x, y, z. Women who will completely starve themselves to look like the – mostly photoshopped – versions of other people instead of becoming the best version of themselves.

If I return to the nature of your hair, the subject of this book, I witnessed the reality of what this kind of behaviour does for the health of your hair. During many tests for my hairbrush line Delphin & Emerence, I had the pleasure to meet women from all colors, shapes and textures. What struck me the most, was that

Embrace your true nature!

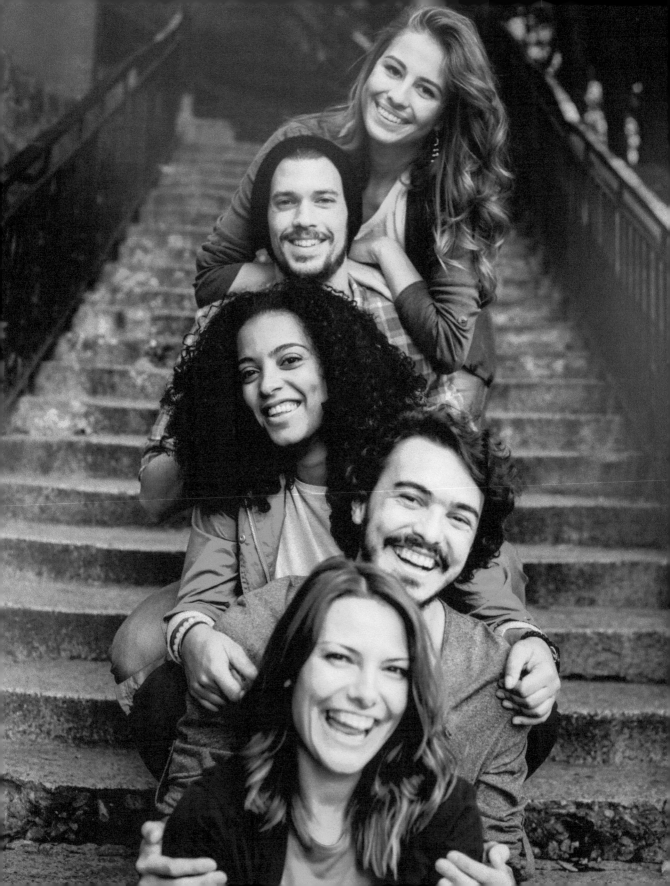

many women, especially the ones with African-American and North-African hair, wanted to change their natural style so drastically with harsh treatments that their hair literally broke upon touching it. I saw ladies with bald spots due to the many aggressive treatments. I witnessed painfully hurt red and dry scalp and I heard of the strangest treatments ever. At some point I was truly shocked to see how all these beautiful women abused their hair because of their desire to achieve that perfect beauty image. I saw all these beautiful girls and ladies and when I asked them if they would like to be a model for the campaign of Delphin & Emerence, they almost all said that they wouldn't participate, because they thought they weren't pretty enough or didn't possess the perfect figure of a model, or this or that... This has touched me very deeply.

That's why I'm so happy that there are positive role models, who love their curves and even make it their trademark. Or the ones who let their natural hair color and texture shine, like Oprah Winfrey did by making her Afro roots rock during her shows and on the cover of *O Magazine*.

Also the singer Erykah Badu and Solange Knowles of *Destiny's Child* made a statement of their natural hair. I know that as a blonde with fine hair, I probably don't have a say in the behaviour of people of different hair textures or how they need to treat it, but I'm very concerned about the well-being of everyone. This is why I couldn't leave this part out of my book.

And by the way, also blondes, redheads, people with loose curls or straight hair, we all have done crazy things to change ourselves, haven't we? My attempt in achieving perfectly brown locks didn't have a beautiful result either. So love yourself, treat yourself well and emphasize what is given to you. This is you and we love you!

HAIR LOSS: WHEN DO YOU HAVE TO BE CONCERNED?

Normally you will lose an average of 50-100 hairs per day. This is perfectly normal and the longer your hair, the more it appears to be in your hairbrush or shower drain. When you lose more hair than normal or when you notice that the loss of hair is speeded up or only affects certain parts of the head, it's best to ask advice from a health care practioner or doctor. Hair loss is a warning sign of our body to tell us that something is wrong. Hormonal imbalance, stress, problems with your thyroid, immune diseases... could be the cause of abnormal hair loss.

Hair loss can occur in different phases of your life and isn't always age-related. To determine if you lose more hair than normal, there are a few signs to pay attention to:

- you see hair on your pillow in the morning

- when you gently brush or pull your hair, hair comes loose more easily than normal.

THE ROLE OF HORMONES AND HAIR GROWTH

The best proof that hormones have an influence on our hair growth can be seen in the differences between men and women, especially in the areas where hair develops on the body. This is the reason why men have a moustache, beard and longer hair on the chest and why women don't have this unless their hormone levels are out of balance.

ROLE OF DHT: DIHYDROTESTOSTERONE

The hormone 'dihydrotestosterone' or DHT is formed from the male hormone testosterone in which the enzyme 5-alpha-reductase plays an important role. DHT isn't only for men, both men and women generate this hormone.

DHT is a hormone that induces hair loss, the so-called 'androgenic alopecia'. In men, this manifests itself in the regression/retraction of the front hairline and balding until this process reaches a final stage with only hair left on the back of the scalp. In women we notice thinning hair on the crown, and after a while you even start to easily 'see' the scalp through the hairs.

How is DHT formed? This process goes on in the hair follicle, remember?

The moment that DHT is going to bind to androgen receptors, it slows the growth phase of the hair and eventually the hair follicle dies, making the hair fall out. If this process continues, you will get more and more hair loss.

Unfortunately it's also a part of getting older. It's going faster in men than in women (sorry guys!). It clearly troubles people, if you notice the amount of commercials made for hair growth products and treatments. However, if you take good care of your hair, eat healthy and take the right vitamins... you can noticeably slow down this process. Though it may not always solve the genetic factors and any underlying health problems.

SALLY GRAY, ND, NATUROPATH - NUTRITIONIST - HERBALIST

"The impact of hormones on the condition of hair is something I see a lot in my practice.
Many women experience dramatic changes with their hair during and after pregnancy due to an increase in the hormone estrogen which prolongs the growth phase of hair allowing for more lustrous locks during pregnancy. When estrogen diminishes after birth, the hair returns to its usual pattern of hair growth and loss. The latter often appears worse with the addition of cortisol, our stress hormone, which often comes into play with a newborn on the scene and our new busier life! Hormonal imbalance can be a common trigger for hair changes and is always an area of investigation in my clinic."

AND WHAT DURING (PERI-)MENOPAUSE?

An expert speaking: Haylie Pomroy, nutritionist and author of *Fast Metabolism Food Rx* and *The Fast Metabolism Diet*.

My good friend Haylie Pomroy explained to me in a simple way, what the peri-menopause and menopause mean for your hair:

"During each major hormone surge, the body enters a phase in which it is looking for a balance between the natural sex hormones estrogen, progesterone and testosterone and the hormone produced in the adrenal glands (cortisol).

Sometimes it happens that in that process the new standard, the new balance does not get settled. For me as a nutritionist the following changes in my patients' hair raise a red flag: brittle hair, dry hair, hair prone to breakage, changes in volume and especially the thinning of the hair at the crown. These are signs to me that there is a hormonal imbalance in the body. That's when I make a customized nutrition and supplementation plan for my clients."

This is you and we love you!

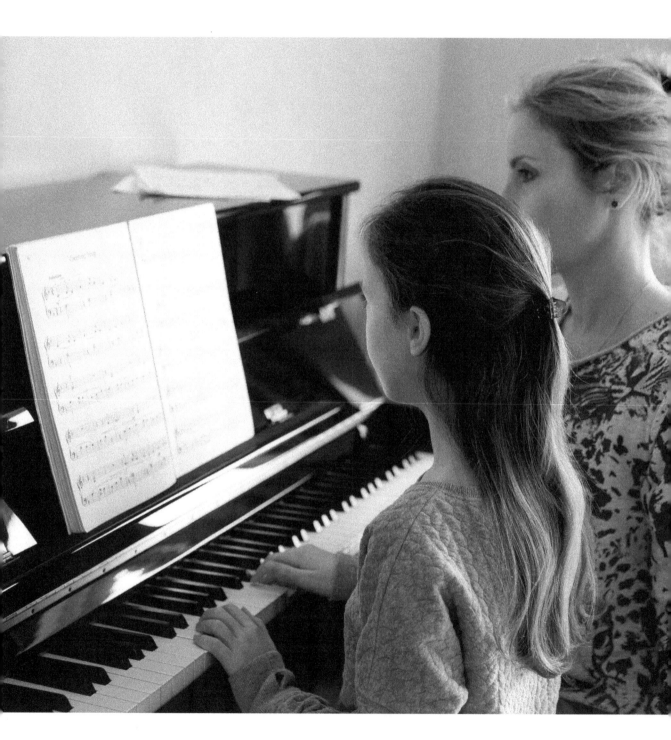

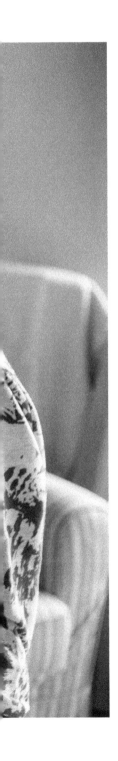

THE INFLUENCE OF THE THYROID

The thyroid or *glandula thyroidea* is a butterfly-shaped gland that is situated on the front side of the neck, around the throat. The thyroid gives the following hormones: T3 (Tri-ioidothyronine) and T4 (Thyroxine).

The thyroid hormones regulate a number of important metabolic and growth processes in the body. Describing the whole process that is being regulated by the thyroid would be too much for this book, but I particularly want to indicate that the thyroid may be one of the possible culprits, if you are experiencing hair problems. It is therefore important that a doctor examines it. When the thyroid function is disrupted, it can result in the production of either too little or too many of its hormones.

Especially during pregnancy this imbalance can happen. Some of the symptoms (depending on a too fast or too slow working thyroid) could be:

- quick and unexplainable **gaining** or **losing body weight**

- extreme **fatigue** and **lethargy** or **overactivity** and **restlessness**

- **hair loss**

- **weak immune system.**

So make sure that when you have persistent hair problems, that you have yourself examined by a medical doctor to rule out thyroid problems. Regulating the thyroid gland can be done with appropriate medication, but there are treatments that help to support your thyroid with a balanced diet and nutritional supplements. So make sure you also ask for these methods of treatment.

OTHER CULPRITS OF HAIR LOSS

Besides the ones listed above, there can be other things that cause hair loss or brittle hair:

- **a lack** of **nutrients**

- **cancer**

- **lupus**

- **immune diseases**

- **stress**

- **birth control:** the type of pill you take, hormones or IUD may be a cause of hair loss

- **diabetes**

- **disturbed blood sugar levels**

- **medication**

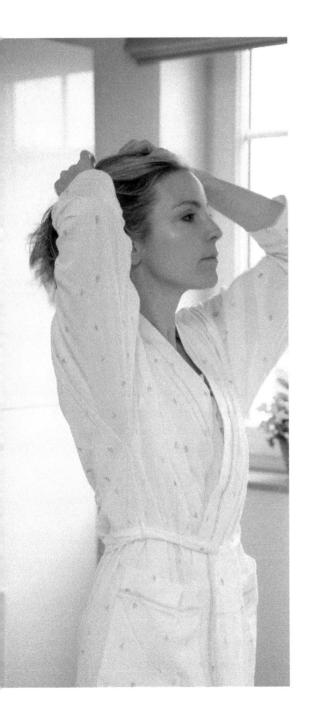

- **mistreating your hair:** too much styling, backcombing, the use of a bad brush, using rubber bands...

- **exposure** to **toxic substances** and **pollution**

- **eating disorders** such as **anorexia nervosa** or **bulimia**.

Make sure you get a medical check-up to rule out any of the above issues. Your hair (and nails) are an important messenger of your body and you should never ignore the signs. Your body wants to tell you something: listen to it!

THE THREE STEPS TO HEALTHY HAIR

All right, you have now become a bit of a hair specialist, but you still doubt how to achieve this healthy head of hair. After years of self-research and self-study about the subject, I came to the conclusion that there isn't just one rule, but three. It's a combination of three basic steps that make sure you can look happily in the mirror every morning.

Actually it is a general rule in health, that it is an 'and-and-story'. We are used to a fast-paced life in the western world where we fail to take time to listen to our body and we want a quick fix for every small ailment. Just a pill or a lotion isn't the solution. It's a combination of certain basic rules and three essential steps, which are being addressed in the next chapters. A small sample of what you can expect in the rest of this book:

STEP 1 > nutrition for your hair

STEP 2 > stress management: Take You Time

STEP 3 > the proper hair care.

NUTRITION FOR YOUR HAIR

The first step in the road to overall health and healthy hair is your nutrition pattern, which should be based on 'real' food. Only wholesome, fresh food is able to provide us with the necessary power to optimally grow our hair. A diet that lacks these whole foods and nutrients, sooner or later has a very profound impact on every aspect of your health. Your hair is one of those.

STRESS MANAGEMENT

Too much stress has an impact on your overall health and your hair. In this chapter I discuss the impact of stress and I give a lot of tips and tricks to deal with it. I will teach you to 'Take You Time'.

THE PROPER HAIR CARE

This is often the first step that one takes when hair problems arise. It is an important step, but not the only one. Together with the two other pillars, proper hair care will support and stimulate its growth, it is the finishing touch in the program. You learn the right tips and tricks to use the right over-the-counter products or home-made remedies straight from Mother Nature to deeply nourish your hair in all softness, to protect it from external influences.

Forget not that the earth delights
to feel your bare feet and the
winds long to play with your hair.

KHALIL GIBRAN

The best

are conceived

thoughts

by brushing.

LIES HELSLOOT

FOOD

FOR

HAIR

In this chapter I will explain the first building block for healthy hair locks: a varied diet, rich in the right quantities of vitamins, minerals, amino acids and fats. 'You are what you eat' also applies to your hair. We often have the urge to handle a hair or skin problem on the outside of our body, with some kind of ointment or treatment, but it's better to work on the problem from the inside out. You can achieve this through food, so that your hair will be provided with the best building materials. Below are some common misconceptions about hair that we will unveil in this chapter:

MISCONCEPTIONS

- My **hair** is **solely broken** due to **bad treatment**, nutrition has nothing to do with that.

- My hair is brittle, I have less hair since **pregnancy** and I'm **getting older**. I just have to accept this, because there is nothing I can do about it.

- I want to **stay thin**, so... **no fats** and **skipping meals** once in a while is the best remedy! It can't hurt my hair when I always apply conditioner.

- A hair is **dead material**, right? How can nutrition change the way it looks?

- Nuts? They only make you fat, right?

"Personal note: "When I attended high school, I did a lot of babysitting to earn some pocket money. The kids in our neighbourhood called my sister and me 'the girls with long hair'. They always asked us for our secret, and we always answered that if they finished their plates and made healthy choices, their hair would be as beautiful and long as ours. Well, it wasn't a lie, girls!"

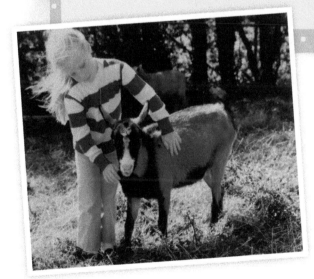

THE IMPORTANCE OF HEALTHY AND BALANCED NUTRITION.

I'm convinced that healthy nutrition, rich in vitamins and minerals, is one of the building blocks of a healthy body and hair. 'You are what you eat' is not a cliché! Our current refined nutrition contains a lot of things we don't need and very little of the things we do need.

Many people with health issues are often searching for quick solutions like a pill, or pass the blame onto their genes, but if you really want to be healthy, you need to face the real reason: your diet.

You could read how a single hair strand is built and what the growth of hair looks like in the first chapter. To support the growth of hair in the most optimal way, you need the right building blocks to grow firm and healthy hair.

Without the right fuel your car won't get far. Healthy hair can be supported and nourished in different ways, but most importantly, healthy hair and health in general come from within.

When we see something on the 'outside' that we don't want to see, like hair problems, we have to ask ourselves the right questions to expose the real problem. Hair problems are signals of your body that something is wrong, this cannot be ignored. A medical specialist, an orthomolecular physician, or a health practitioner who digs deep enough and has enough knowledge and passion to look beyond the obvious, can help you with this by taking a good look at your eating and living habits.

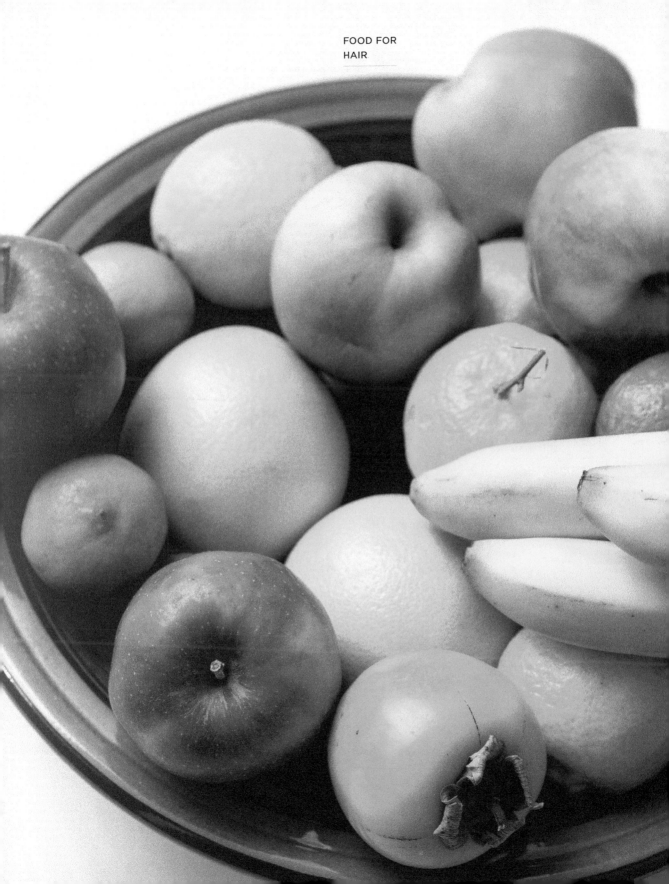

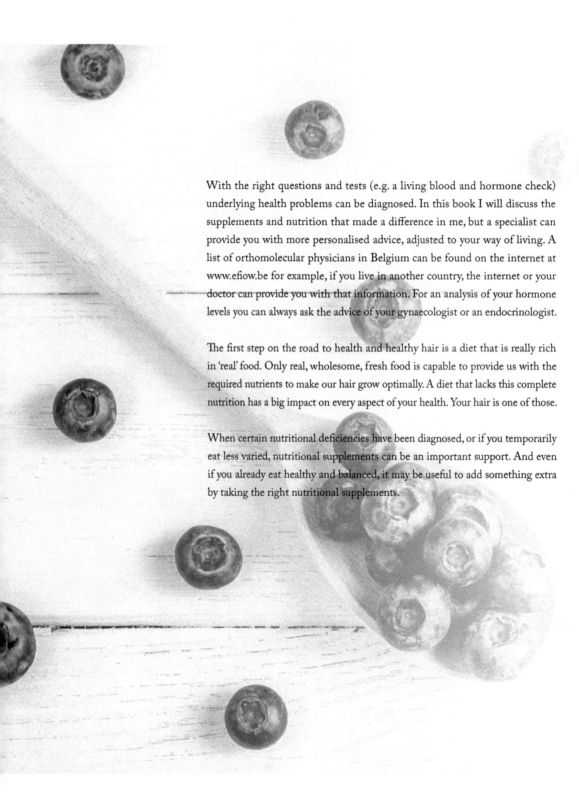

With the right questions and tests (e.g. a living blood and hormone check) underlying health problems can be diagnosed. In this book I will discuss the supplements and nutrition that made a difference in me, but a specialist can provide you with more personalised advice, adjusted to your way of living. A list of orthomolecular physicians in Belgium can be found on the internet at www.efiow.be for example, if you live in another country, the internet or your doctor can provide you with that information. For an analysis of your hormone levels you can always ask the advice of your gynaecologist or an endocrinologist.

The first step on the road to health and healthy hair is a diet that is really rich in 'real' food. Only real, wholesome, fresh food is capable to provide us with the required nutrients to make our hair grow optimally. A diet that lacks this complete nutrition has a big impact on every aspect of your health. Your hair is one of those.

When certain nutritional deficiencies have been diagnosed, or if you temporarily eat less varied, nutritional supplements can be an important support. And even if you already eat healthy and balanced, it may be useful to add something extra by taking the right nutritional supplements.

ABOUT SUPPLEMENTS

Choose premium brands when you buy vitamins. Good brands are more expensive than inferior brands, but contain more of the good quality vitamins. These premium brands contain a better ratio of vitamins so your body can absorb them better. Brands like Life Extension (the best!) and Pharma Nord have been offering the best quality for years. When you take a multivitamin preparation, you will get a lot of the vitamins that are listed below. It isn't necessary to add more of the same vitamins in a separate supplement.

There are also preparations on the market that are specifically designed for your hair and nails. Good brands are Oenobiol, Phyto, Innéov and supplements targeting hormonal problems , like 'Metabolism T4T3' developed by Haylie Pomroy.

AN EXPERT SPEAKING:
HAYLIE POMROY, NUTRITIONIST

"In my practice, nutrition is the most important medicine to optimize the health of my clients. With my female clients I often see hair loss after pregnancy because of the stress the body undergoes during childbirth. In order to achieve a new balance in the body various therapies may be used of which the provision of the right foods rich in enzymes and phytonutrients forms the basis. I write a natural, sometimes macrobiotic diet plan and make use of what nature provides by introducing for example maca, turmeric, green tea and spirulina for their anti-inflammatory and antioxidant properties. Hair growth is, after all, a process of fast-growing cells, and such nutrients ensure that the hair cells do not die in an early phase of growth, so hair loss can be avoided."

EAT!

Do not starve yourself! I do not believe in skipping meals. I did it too often in the past when in a rush and time constrained, I just forgot to eat. I often see this pattern with women who think this is the way to stay thin. What concerns me most is that young girls, whose bodies are not yet fully grown, try to apply these techniques to fit into a size zero. So they can 'fit in', incited by photoshopped role models in magazines and on television. By not eating you will drain your body in the long term, something I experienced myself. It does have a negative effect on your hair. I'm not talking about fasting once in a while because of health reasons, detox or religious reasons. Fasting can have a set place in those situations, but I've learned to eat regularly. I eat a healthy breakfast, healthy lunch and dinner and as a snack I eat a handful of nuts, a piece of fruit or a healthy smoothie with fruits or vegetables. I really had to learn to include healthy snacks, but I was encouraged by my friend Haylie Pomroy, a nutritionist, to do so.

A healthy plate consists of a lot of vegetables in all the colours of the rainbow. I usually choose whole grains, eat a lot of legumes and I'm not afraid of an extra spoon of extra virgin olive oil. I make sure my menus are rich in protein. To compose a healthy plate, I personally think the Sana-principles of Sandra Bekkari are very useful and clear. The books of Haylie Pomroy also contain balanced meal plans with delicious and simple recipes. Other fun and healthy books are those of:

· Gwyneth Paltrow, It's All Easy: Delicious Weekday Recipes for the Super-Busy Home Cook

· Martha Stewart, Power Foods: 150 Delicious Recipes with the 38 Healthiest Ingredients

· Jamie Oliver, Everyday Super Food and Super Food Family Classics

· Pascale Naessens: all her books are good for delicious and healthy cooking

· Rens Kroes (a Dutch health foodie and sister of Doutzen Kroes).

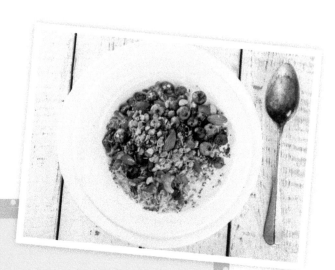

PERSONAL TIP

I usually start my day with a bowl full of organic Greek yoghurt and lots of fresh fruit and berries (frozen or fresh) topped with some seeds and two to four spoons of natural unsweetened muesll with oatmeal. I combine this with 100 ml of my self-made cocktail of pure juice in a mixture of equal parts of blueberry, pomegranate and cranberry juice.

I always go for non-diluted juices without extra-added sugar from the health food store. To make it a bit less sour I add a few drops of stevia extract. This berry cocktail is filled with antioxidants and anthocyanins that counter the ageing process. I'm convinced after years that this is a good habit, which affects my health in general.

SALLY GRAY, NATUROPATH, NUTRITIONIST AND HERBALIST:

"Your nutrition plan needs to be focussed on high quality, 'real' food and wholesome ingredients. Avoid refined and overprocessed food."

More information on Sally Gray on: www.sallygraynd.com

Avoid refined and processed foods.

PROTEÏNS

A hair is build from keratin, which is a protein. That's why it is of great importance that protein is a part of your diet. I myself thought that I was eating healthy, because I was eating a vegetarian diet with mostly vegetables, fruit and whole grains, but I forgot to add protein on a regular basis.

Consequently, my hair condition worsened, I lost muscle mass and I was often tired and suffered one cold after another. Too little protein makes your hair dry, brittle and weak. Extreme deficiencies in protein can cause hair loss. Now I do pay attention to add sufficient proteins to my meals.

YOU CAN FIND HEALTHY PROTEINS IN:

* **poultry** (chicken, turkey...)

* **fish:** make sure you don't skip the fatty fish types, which are full of omega 3 and are extra healthy for your hair. Two birds with one stone!

* **natural yoghurt** (I eat my Greek yoghurt on a daily basis)

* **eggs**

- **lean meat:** in moderation. Reserve it for special occasions. Consuming meat, especially red meat, is not the wisest choice in general. Scientists have shown that eating red meat increases the production of DHT (dihydrotestosteron). DHT makes our hair thinner and leads to rapid hair loss.

- **nuts** (almonds, walnuts, hazelnuts, brazil nuts...)

- **legumes** (peas, lentils, chickpeas, white beans, borlottl beans...)

- **tofu** and **tempeh**, both made from soybeans.

Some people believe that taking keratin supplements makes your hair stronger. I don't have any experience with this, but after reading up on the subject, I have some concerns about it. Since the low-carb trend, in which people eliminated carbohydrates, and often only ate large quantities of protein, doctors and health coaches became worried about the impact on our health.

Low-carb protein diets definitely have their value, if they are used for short periods under supervision of specialists to speed up weight loss. Our body can't process a large supply of protein in the long term. The kidneys, which drain the surplus of protein, need to work extra hard to process them and this can cause kidney problems. I can recommend you to consult a specialist or an orthomo-lecular doctor to ask for advice. Supplements with extra keratin are also a form of protein supplements, hence my caveat.

OMEGA 3

This exceptional nutrient became popular about fifteen years ago. And with good reason! I got to know this substance through Jo Wyckmans during the years that I worked in my health food restaurant.

This man spoke so passionately about the role and power of omega 3 that you had to become a believer. He wrote a great book on it – *Healthy on the inside, beautiful on the outside* – and from his passion for health and his perfectionism, he created a series of supplements named 'Minami Nutrition'. He witnessed, during his life in the fashion world, how super thin models denied themselves very important nutrients, by following completely crazy and wrong diets, which created a shortage of omega 3.

Our body can't produce omega 3 itself. It is very important that we gain this nutrient through our food. Omega 3 fatty acids are located in the cells in the scalp and supply our body with the necessary building blocks to make natural skin oils, which keep the scalp and hair hydrated.

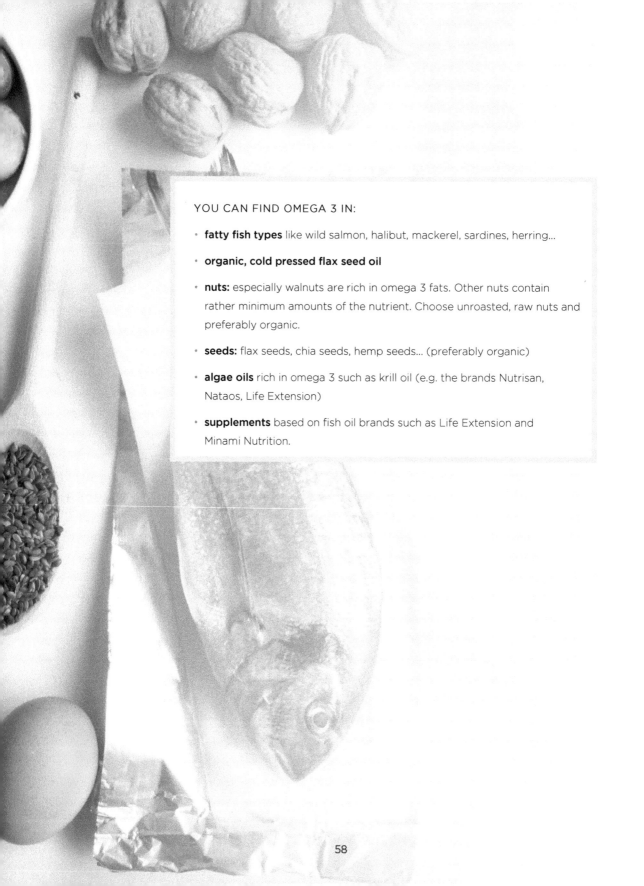

YOU CAN FIND OMEGA 3 IN:

- **fatty fish types** like wild salmon, halibut, mackerel, sardines, herring...

- **organic, cold pressed flax seed oil**

- **nuts:** especially walnuts are rich in omega 3 fats. Other nuts contain rather minimum amounts of the nutrient. Choose unroasted, raw nuts and preferably organic.

- **seeds:** flax seeds, chia seeds, hemp seeds... (preferably organic)

- **algae oils** rich in omega 3 such as krill oil (e.g. the brands Nutrisan, Nataos, Life Extension)

- **supplements** based on fish oil brands such as Life Extension and Minami Nutrition.

TIPS FROM NUTRITIONIST
HAYLIE POMROY

"To restore the hormonal balance in your body, healthy fats in your diet are very important. The reason for this is that they are precursors of our hormones. In addition, all foods that support the liver are of critical importance, such as onions, garlic and so-called cruciferous vegetables like broccoll and cabbages. The reason is that these foods contain phytonutrients and plant-based enzymes that help the body in the conversion of hormones. Thus, the balance can be restored."

More information on Haylie Pomroy at www.hayliepomroy.com

L-LYSINE

L-Lysine is an amino acid that is often prescribed for the treatment of hair loss. It is also a powerful tool in the prevention and healing of cold sores. You can find it as a supplement with the better brands. You can find it in the following foods: cheese, yoghurt, fish and soy products.

VITAMIN C

Linus Pauling, considered by many as the founder of orthomolecular medicine, began researching the link between the right proportions of vitamins in the body back in the sixties along with his assistant Paul Staunton. He was particularly passionate about the influence of vitamin C.

Vitamin C is an important antioxidant and is rapidly consumed by the body. Vitamin C helps in the production of collagen in the connective tissues necessary for inter alia healthy skin and hair, and strengthens the capillaries that supply the follicles with the right nutrients.

The best natural sources of vitamin C are blackcurrants, blueberries, broccoli, guava, kiwi, oranges, papaya, strawberries, sweet potatoes... Someone who's on a good diet with lots of fresh fruit and vegetables, alternating between raw and cooked food, basically has enough vitamin C to withstand attacks from the outside and to build a good immune system.

Vitamin C is very rapidly consumed and excreted by the body, it won't be stored. In our society, in which we are confronted with pollution, bacteria and viruses, our bodies can use some extra help.

I take vitamin C as a supplement every day in the form of 'buffered' vitamin C, even though I also eat a lot of vegetables and fruit. For years I have been using the buffered vitamin C from the brand *Life Extension*, which sells top quality supplements.

My skin looks more fresh and firm, wrinkles diminished (more collagen), my hair grows healthy again and I rarely get sick. And when I'm sick, I quickly get better due to the extra vitamin C. I take vitamin C until my body reaches a satisfaction level, that's the point where your stool is getting very thin. For myself it's around an intake of five to seven grams of 'buffered' vitamin C.

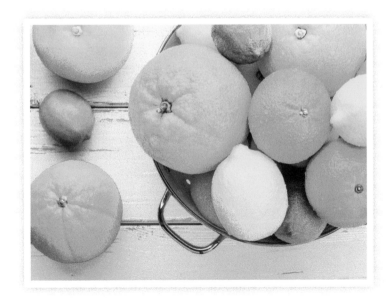

NO SMOKING!

No smoking for smoking hot hair! That should be your motto. Smoking is bad for your general health and the people around you. But did you know that smoking gives you wrinkles and causes a faint complexion? And did you know that it has a negative impact on your hair?

Smoking causes your body to absorb less oxygen, which is needed for the oxygen supply to the skin and hair. Carbon monoxide instead of oxygen is then transported to your cells and the supply of blood, rich of nutrients, is prevented so your hair won't receive the needed nutrition from within.

VITAMIN A

Our body needs vitamin A to make sebum in the sebaceous glands. This sebum is, as explained in chapter 1, your natural conditioner for healthy hair and scalp. Without sebum we would have a very dry and itchy scalp and dry hair. Make sure you put enough animal products on the menu that are rich in this vitamin, like liver . Besides that, you can choose orange and yellow vegetables and fruits (carrots, pumpkins, paprikas, sweet potatoes, kakis) with a high content of beta-carotene, which provides for the production of vitamin A.

VITAMINS FROM THE B-GROUP

For general health, all B-vitamins are essential in the right proportions. Amongst this group are different kinds, that are not only good for healthy hair growth, but that also support your body in some vital processes and support you in stressful situations. A good multivitamin (for example the 'Life Extension Mix' or 'Two-per-day tablets') will offer you the full spectrum of B-vitamins, but your diet remains the most important and primary source.

The following vitamins are part of the B-group: B1 (thiamine), B2 (riboflavin), B3 (niacin), B5 (pantothenic acid), B6 (pyridoxine), B7 (biotin), B9 (folic acid) and B12. Biotin is a water-soluble vitamin and is often added to hair vitamins, although all the other B vitamins remain equally important. When you don't ingest enough biotin in your diet, you get very brittle, weak hair and possibly also hair loss. Make sure you get enough biotin from eating: whole grains, liver, egg yolks, soy flour and yeast (e.g. yeast powder from the health food store).

IRON

Iron is a very important mineral for hair growth. If you have low iron levels (anaemia), this may be an important factor in hair loss. The hair follicle and the hair root are both fed by a nutrient-rich blood supply. When the iron level (serum ferritin) goes below a certain point, you can get anaemia. This process disrupts the nutrient supply to the follicle and affects the hair growth cycle negatively and can eventually result in hair loss.

Animal products such as red meat, liver, egg yolks, nuts, beans, oats, oysters, chicken and fish provide your body iron in a well absorbable form, making it easily and immediately available to support the body processes. When you eat a vegetarian diet, as was my case, you should definitely pay attention to get enough iron by adding lentils, spinach and other green leafy vegetables (broccoli, kale, salad) to your diet. Also provide a combination of iron-rich foods with vitamin C, because this vitamin promotes the absorption of iron.

ZINC AND SELENIUM

Zinc and selenium are very important substances for your overall health: they support your immune system, make your hair and nails grow stronger and help to maintain a healthy skin. Selenium also plays a role in the normal functioning of the thyroid gland and may therefore support to achieve optimal hormone levels. Zinc is often prescribed to boost your immune system as it helps to prevent viruses to bind to the lining of your nose, helping to prevent you from getting a cold. Zinc also ensures an optimal production of T-cells, the 'fighter cells' in our immune system.

You can ensure to incorporate them into your daily diet or you can take them in the form of a good multivitamin (e.g. 'Two-per-day', *Life Extension* or 'Life Extension Mix'). There are also preparations to take this nutrient separately, for example 'Selenium + Zinc' *Pharma Nord* and 'Super Selenium Complex' and 'Zinc Caps' from *Life Extension*.

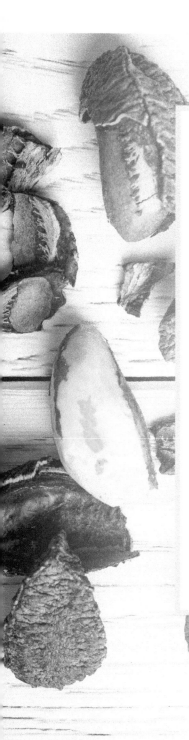

You can find zinc and selenium, among others, in the following food sources:

- **brazil nuts**

- **oysters,**

- **spinach**

- **wheat germ**

- **eggs**

- **beef**

- **lamb**

- **black chocolate** (preferably raw and/or at least 70% cocoa content)

- **cocoa powder** (preferably raw)

- **cashews**

- **pumpkin seeds...**

...

For example, a daily dose of one or two Brazil nuts is sufficient to provide your body with the necessary selenium. It is nevertheless recommended not to eat more than six pieces of this kind of nut because you will receive an overload of this micronutrient. This can lead to abdominal pain, fatigue, brittle nails, itching and skin rashes.

If you are in doubt about overdosing, ask advice from a specialised nutritionist with knowledge about orthomolecular nutritional medicine.

MSM

MSM (methylsulfonylmethane) is an organic sulphur compound consisting of sulphur and methyl groups. The substance is naturally found in plants, animals and humans. As a dietary supplement, MSM became popular in the last ten years as a natural pain reliever and as support for problems with the musculoskeletal system such as arthritis, rheumatism, muscle cramps, injuries in sports, wound healing, fibromyalgia and lower back pain...

MSM is also used successfully in the treatment of allergies (hay fever and asthma). MSM improves the absorption of minerals, vitamins and amino acids and is known for its rejuvenating properties. It is widely hailed in the books of raw food guru David Wolfe.

The food also has a nice extra: it's very beneficial for the growth of hair and nails, which is why it absolutely had to be described in this book.

You can find MSM in foods high in protein such as eggs, meat, poultry and fish. It is also found in seafood and onions.

TIP

"I myself take MSM every day, in tablet form (Life Extension) or an oral solution ('Dexsil Forte', which also contains silicon, chondroitin and glucosamine). If I do not take it for a few weeks, I notice an immediate effect on my hair growth and firmness of my nails. For me it's a top winner for my hair and nails."

SILICON

Silicon is an important building block of the connective tissue and plays a role in the synthesis of collagen and keratin, two substances that have an influence on hair growth and firm skin.

A better quality collagen ensures healthy hair growth and a strong hair shaft. Organically bound silicon can support this process and help prevent hair loss. Silicon helps to keep the collagen in the blood vessels around the hair follicles smooth and supple. You can take additional silicon in supplement form, but always make sure that it's organically bound silicon, which is better absorbed by your body. Good brands include: *Dexsil, Biosil, Hübner.* There are also lotions and balms based on silicon, to apply as a topical external treatment.

RESVERATROL

Resveratrol is a natural ingredient, polyphenol, found in various plants, but especially in the peel of grapes. It is the substance that gives grapevines a natural protection against the daily influence of the weather and protects the plant against fungI among others . Because of these properties, scientists were curious to investigate what this substance can do for our health.

Many studies have shown that resveratrol has a rejuvenating effect on the body and that it is a powerful weapon in the prevention of cancer.

IN A BOOK WRITTEN BY
DOCTORS RICHARD BÉLIVEAU AND
DENIS GINGRAS, IT IS DESCRIBED AS FOLLOWS:

"Thus, resveratrol is one of the herbal ingredients with the strongest anti-cancer effect and may prevent both the onset and progression of cancer... Through this process the concentrations of resveratrol that we receive from a moderate consumption of red wine would be enough to intervene in the development of cancer, especially when the wine is made from grapes that contain significant amounts of the molecule, especially the pinot noir." (Source: Preventing Cancer, Reducing The Risks, Richard Béliveau and Denis Gingras, 2015, Kosmos Publishers, ISBN-10: 1770856331, ISBN-13: 978-1770856332)

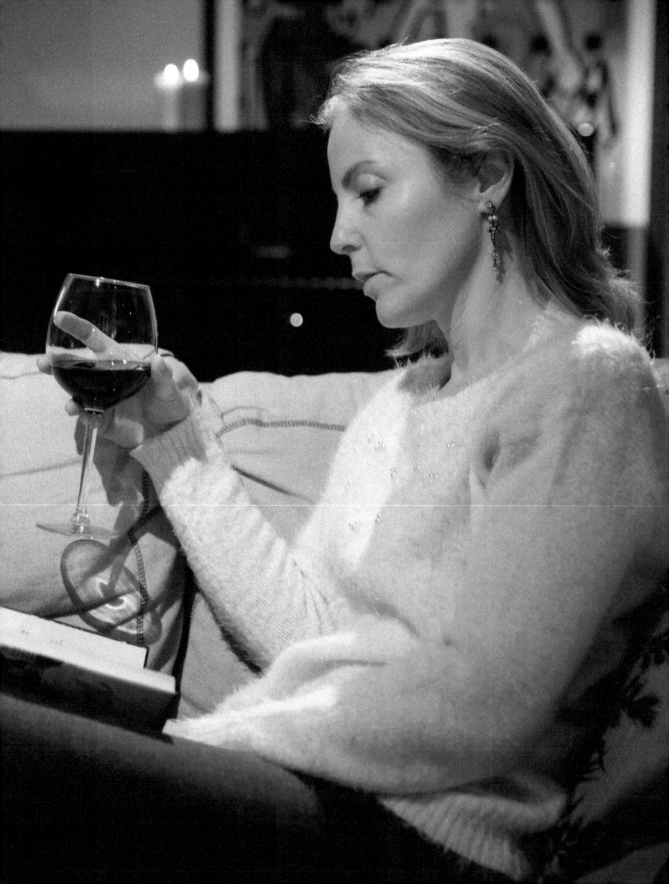

Resveratrol also has rejuvenating properties and a strong antioxidant action thereby addressing inflammation and it protects our body against the processes related with aging and the impact of UVA radiation. It ensures that collagen levels are maintained, allowing your skin to be fresh, healthy and less wrinkled. Therefore it is also beneficial for healthy hair because the scalp is kept in optimum condition.

It is currently used in skin care products, with the French brand Caudalie at the top of the list successfully adding the substance to their range of products, so that it can optimally work its magic on the skin.

Do you need more resveratrol in your diet? Drink a regular glass of good red wine with high resveratrol content. Especially Pinot Noir from areas in Australia and France (Loire, Bourgogne) have a particularly high resveratrol content (Source: *Preventing Cancer, Reducing The Risks*, Richard Béliveau and Denis Gingras, 2015, Kosmos Publishers, ISBN-10: 1770856331, ISBN-13: 978-1770856332)

However, this is not an argument for more alcohol, I am talking about the protective effect of the substances in red wine in case of moderate consumption. The recommendations for alcohol consumption clearly indicate that a daily consumption of alcohol is best restricted to two drinks for men and one for women (source: American Cancer Society). Consuming more alcohol can lead to addiction and the promotion of certain types of cancer. For example, I have a habit to drink a glass of red wine several times per week, but it does not have to be a full glass, I usually limit myself to half a glass.

If, for some reason, you do not wish to consume alcohol, you can find resveratrol in supplement form with brands like *Life Extension* and *Caudalie*. As a dietary supplement resveratrol is particularly powerful in the fight against the aging process.

VITAMIN E

Vitamin E is a fat-soluble vitamin and a powerful antioxidant that helps to protect your hair and skin against the harmful effects of the sun. Therefore, it is important to include sufficient amounts of vitamin E in the diet. Vitamin E is found in nuts, wheat germ oil, organic whole wheat flour, wheat germs (organic), eggs, …

It is also a powerful cure against the ageing of the skin, because it slows the cell ageing process. A bonus, right?

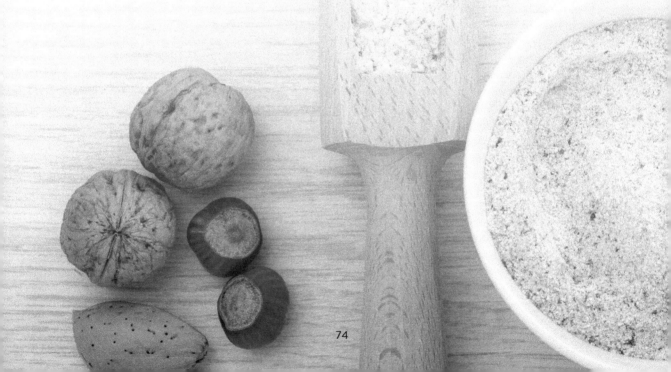

*This is you and
we love you!*

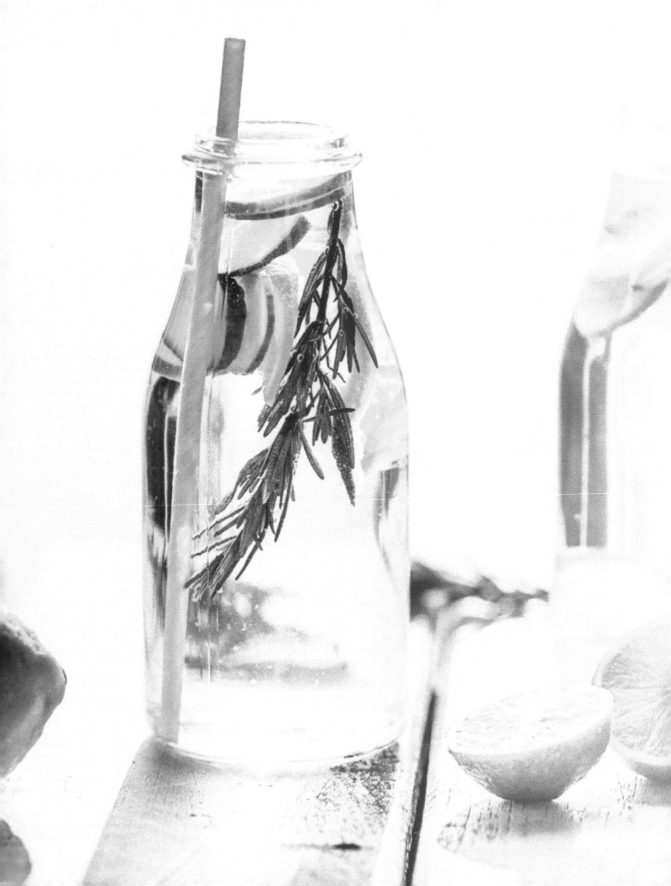

WATER: THE HEALTHY THIRST QUENCHER AND SOURCE OF LIFE.

Yeah, I know, you say. Yet a reminder to drink water now and then is a must. Drinking water is very important. It hydrates your skin, gets rid of toxins, clears your head and it also provides for a healthy head of hair.

Drink one and a half to two liters of water per day, preferably filtered water (to minimize your carbon footprint, such as a *Brita* filter for your water jug or a reverse osmosis filter on your tap) or mineral water with a low dry residue content, good brands include *Mont Roucous, Lifjalla, Spa Reine, Evian...*

Do you like to drink something with a flavour? You could try homemade ice tea without sugar, or water with a few slices of lime or lemon. Do you prefer something warm, then replace a glass of water with herbal tea. Sodas, even the ones with sugar replacements, absolutely do not belong in a healthy diet.

CRACK A NUT

I mentioned several times the importance of nuts in your diet. Nuts are a healthy snack, contain protein and are packed with healthy nutrients. And eating nuts will not make you fat. I regularly eat a handful of mixed nuts and often add them to salads or other dishes.

I usually carry a jar of nuts in my handbag on days when I'm away from home. That way a healthy snack is always close by. My daughter made it a habit to add this to her menu and takes a box of mixed nuts and dried fruits with her to school.

While writing this book, I wore dental braces which made 'snacking' on nuts and seeds not very easy, as they were 'deliciously' getting stuck between all blocks and wires, therefore I often processed them into them smoothies.

SEA VEGETABLES

Dulse, wakame, nori, hijiki... all healthy gifts from the sea.

They are, easy to digest, low-calorie and rich in different nutrients: iron, iodine, protein, magnesium, potassium, phosphorus, vitamin A, vitamin C... You can find them in any good health food store and nowadays also in supermarkets.

YOUR DAILY CUP OF GREEN TEA

I learned about the pleasure and the benefits of matcha green tea from the Belgian nutritionist Sandra Bekkari. Since then I am a loyal fan. It also gives me the perfect boost, better than coffee, during a busy day. I mix it often with some soy milk for a 'matcha latte'.

I prefer matcha green tea to other types, because it pleases me more in taste and other types often feel heavy on the stomach and make me nauseous. I notice that other people experience the same and since they have discovered matcha, they are adding it to their menu. If you really don't like the taste, you can mix it in a smoothie, fruit juice or a 'matcha latte' with almond or soy milk.

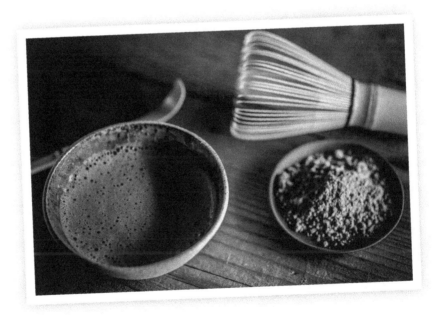

HERBS AND HERBAL MEDICINE FOR YOUR HAIR

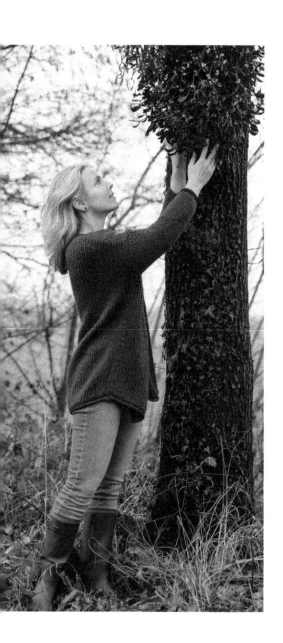

Not only vitamins and minerals are good for your hair, but also the wonderful world of herbs can help you get and maintain a healthy head of hair.

In addition to a healthy diet, you can make sure to include specific nutrients from the rich world of plants and herbs. Mother Nature has a cupboard full of goods. From childhood on, I was fascinated by nature and its variety in the kingdom of plants, the colours and especially the smells and flavours.

As a child I was usually to be found in the woods, near the pond, the many streams in those times where still full of stick-lebacks, or in the meadows around my former home in the paradise-like countryside of the village of Wortegem-Petegem.

We lived on a beautifully restored old farm where my father and mother indulged in their passions during their free time: my dad was responsible for a so-called self-sufficient veg-etable garden and an orchard based on the principles from the books of John Seymour, he bred his own chickens, tur-keys, ducks, sheep, bees... so we always had a good supply of healthy fruits and vegetables, honey from our own bees and meat from animals that were living a nice life and were able to graze freely in our meadows.

Our animals were treated with respect and love, and at the end of their lives, slaughtered on the farm using techniques handed over from father to son, in which my father was always assisted by a - to my feelings as child - very old man

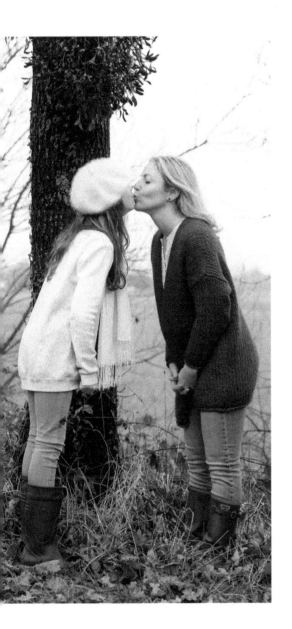

with a blue overcoat. This man still used butcher techniques handed over from father to son with respect for the animal.

Because I experienced the slaughtering process myself, I developed a great respect and gratitude for animals, because I saw with my own eyes that the piece of meat on my plate came from our own animals, raised on our land, and not from a package at the butcher's or supermarket. Nothing was thrown away when killing an animal: the wool of the sheep was processed to knitting wool, sheep skin became leather and the intestines of the animals where being processed into many of my mother's savoury dishes such as pâtés and stews.

While my dad, wearing boots and carrying a shovel, worked the land, my mom was busy milking her goat 'Triene'. The milk was processed into delicious cheeses and other recipes. I always thought it was blissful to help with the milking and vividly remember the smell of the stable, the feel of the soft udders in my hands, the special smell and taste of the goat and the process of cheesemaking.

All of these childhood experiences are also the reason why, while creating my hairbrush line *Delphin & Emerence*, I paid a great deal of attention to natural materials and respect for the welfare of the animals that give me the hair for my brushes. I thank them from the bottom of my heart. I'm not a daily or big meat consumer, but when eating a piece of meat or cheese, I feel the link with the origin of it all and I still say: "thank you."

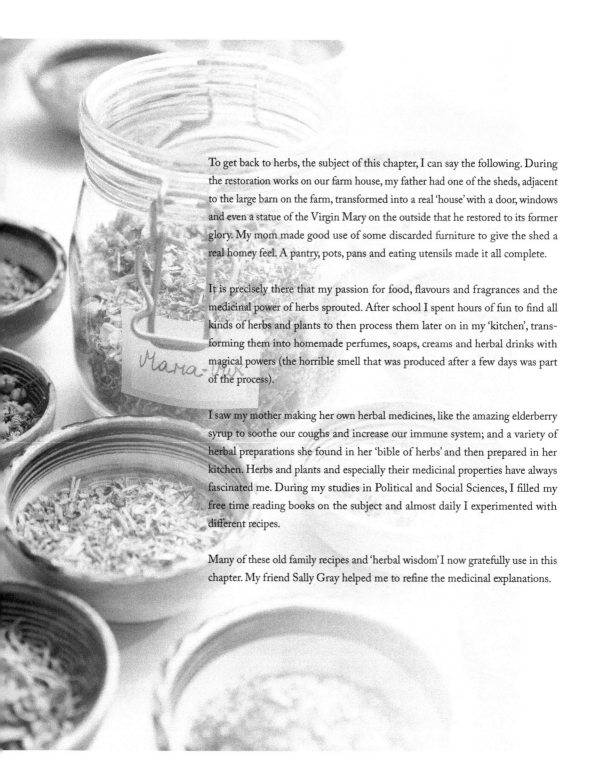

To get back to herbs, the subject of this chapter, I can say the following. During the restoration works on our farm house, my father had one of the sheds, adjacent to the large barn on the farm, transformed into a real 'house' with a door, windows and even a statue of the Virgin Mary on the outside that he restored to its former glory. My mom made good use of some discarded furniture to give the shed a real homey feel. A pantry, pots, pans and eating utensils made it all complete.

It is precisely there that my passion for food, flavours and fragrances and the medicinal power of herbs sprouted. After school I spent hours of fun to find all kinds of herbs and plants to then process them later on in my 'kitchen', transforming them into homemade perfumes, soaps, creams and herbal drinks with magical powers (the horrible smell that was produced after a few days was part of the process).

I saw my mother making her own herbal medicines, like the amazing elderberry syrup to soothe our coughs and increase our immune system; and a variety of herbal preparations she found in her 'bible of herbs' and then prepared in her kitchen. Herbs and plants and especially their medicinal properties have always fascinated me. During my studies in Political and Social Sciences, I filled my free time reading books on the subject and almost daily I experimented with different recipes.

Many of these old family recipes and 'herbal wisdom' I now gratefully use in this chapter. My friend Sally Gray helped me to refine the medicinal explanations.

WE WILL DISCUSS SOME OF THEM HERE:

HORSETAIL

The botanical, Latin name of this plant is *equisetum arvense*. Popularly called the 'ponytail' because it looks like a ponytail swaying. It is a plant that I often played with in my childhood, because you can disassemble the stem into 'cubes'. You should try this yourself. This plant, which is called a weed by many people, has a lot of advantages.

It's rich in silicon (or silicic acid), a substance that provides for stronger hair, good hair growth and reduces hair loss. It also has a lot of other phytotherapeutic benefits on your skin (away go those wrinkles), nails, joints, tendons and muscles because it strengthens the connective tissues and helps to purify the body.

You can consume it through nutritional supplements and you can use it to make herbal tea. For a hair tonic, take two tablespoons of the dried herb and let that seep for about twenty minutes in a little bit of hot water. Filter this mixture and press out the moisture.

Mix this powerful herbal tonicum into a natural hair mask or conditioner, massage it into damp hair and leave it on for half an hour. Meanwhile enjoy a cup of tea made with this herb.

At home I have my special 'mommy-mix', a herbal mix with this herb among others. Delicious with a spoonful of raw, organic honey. Do this weekly for good results. Curious about my 'mommy-mix'? Then quickly go to the last chapter.

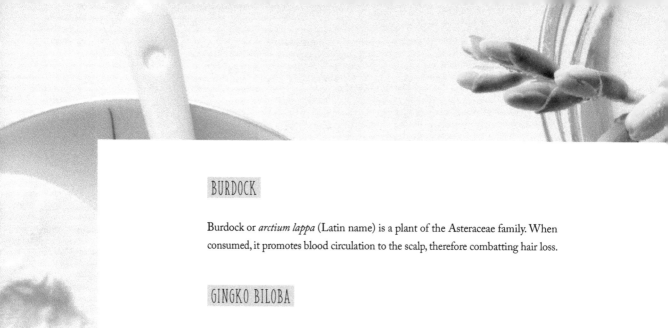

BURDOCK

Burdock or *arctium lappa* (Latin name) is a plant of the Asteraceae family. When consumed, it promotes blood circulation to the scalp, therefore combatting hair loss.

GINGKO BILOBA

Is a herb that is derived from a tree called 'gingko biloba'. A very special, beautiful tree with beautiful leaves. Extracts of this plant contribute to a better condition of and blood circulation in the scalp. Therefore it helps to maintain healthy hair. It is also often used for the support of brain and memory function. Always ask for standardized extracts when you buy medicines based on herbs. A pharmacist with the right knowledge can certainly help you with that.

LARGE NETTLE

The common/stinging nettle or *urtica dioica* is a plant with many uses. Annoying when you are running into it and get stung, but this plant offers so much more: you can eat it like spinach, processed in a healthy spring soup, in cheese, in fantastic tempura or you can make a cup of tea from it. The plant is very effective as a purifying tea and it has a proven effect on hair growth. The plant is rich in iron, silicon, magnesium and calcium, thereby contributing to strong hair.

You can pick them fresh in nature (gloves!!) and in spring when the young nettle shoots are at their best in terms of nutritional content and taste. Definitely pick them from a pesticide-free place. Or visit a good health food store and buy a dried version of the herb. For me it is always an ingredient in my own 'mommy-mix' tea blend. There are also capsules containing extract of the 'common nettle'.

Externally the 'common nettle' was previously being used mainly for the treatment of various hair ailments such as greasy hair, dandruff and lice.

ALOE VERA

Aloe vera stimulates hair growth, promotes circulation and regulates the pH value of the scalp. It can be used externally as a hair mask and is also the best sunburn cure. During the summer months, I always have a bottle in the refrigerator to refresh my skin after a sunny, hot day in open air.

If you wish to take aloe vera internally to strengthen your body, be sure you go for a biological, micro pulp version and keep in mind that aloe vera can have a laxative effect. For internal use, contact an experienced and skilled doctor familiar with alternative therapies or a qualified health practitioner.

THE POWER OF ESSENTIAL OILS

I'm a big fan of essential oils. I always keep them in my home pharmacy and in my handbag. Especially in my travel bag I carry a multi-purpose essential oil mix from the brand *Pranarom* and different capsules from the brand *Primrose*. (when travelling, I have helped many travel companions) It is the healthiest way to keep the indoor air fresh and virus free. You can vaporize the oil in a special diffuser (never over a flame) or you can drizzle a few drops in your vacuum cleaner bag so that you spread a delicious scent around when vacuuming.

There are several essential oils that have a healing effect on hair growth. For example rosemary, lavender and peppermint are known to do this. They can be processed into an oil mix and then massaged into the hair or incorporated in a hair tonic. You can find essential oils at a good pharmacy, health food store or on the internet, for example at www.youngliving.com. Good brands for essential oils include *Pranarom* and *Young Living*. The latter companies also have a range of hair care products that are enriched with the power of essential oils.

Essential oils always have to be diluted before being used on the skin. It is also advisable to be careful using them during pregnancy. It is necessary to provide an adjusted and appropriate dose for children and babies. Please ask for advice from a pharmacist with expertise in this area or a phytotherapist.

Weleda has an excellent hair tonic 'Revitalizing hair lotion' and 'Nourishing Hair Oil' (with rosemary and burdock). Also *Dr. Hauschka* has a hair lotion and hair oil with essential oils , 'Neem Hair Lotion' and 'Neem Hair Oil'. The brand *Phyto* also has a fantastic product called 'Phytopolléine', a useful treatment for those who don't want to prepare their own remedies.

HELP! DO I NEED TO TAKE ALL OF THAT?

The essence

In this chapter we addressed so many things, that it probably overwhelmed you. To give you guidance on your way to a hair-friendly diet, I give a brief checklist with the most important things, so you can check it every day and tick off all the boxes.

THESE ARE THE RULES I FOLLOW MYSELF ON AN EVERYDAY BASIS:

- a healthy breakfast

- two healthy snacks, such as a combination of nuts and fruit

- a lunch and dinner consisting of a variety of colours and flavours, lots of fresh vegetables and a serving of healthy protein

- a daily multivitamin supplement (see recommended brands) provides you with most of the hair-friendly vitamins and minerals described in this chapter

- additionally: 2,000-5,000 mg of buffered vitamin C and a supplement containing MSM

- 1.5 liters of pure water

- a delicious cup of herbal tea from the prescribed herbs (see the recipe for my 'mommy- mix' in the back)

- 1 to 2 cups of green matcha tea

- a daily serving of healthy fats: I take a spoonful of flaxseed oil or an omega 3 supplement every day.

- If a nutritionist or (orthomolecular) doctor prescribed you something extra, of course you must follow his or her directions.

- Still hungry for more tips to feed your hair? Go take a look at my blog www.takeyoutime.com

HAIR–CARE

LIST OF QUESTIONS TO THINK ABOUT:

- I recognize a good shampoo by '**the more foam, the better**'

- **brushing** your hair will **break and damage** your hair

- oh, that **plastic hairbrush** from the supermarket is just as good as an expensive one.

- I **wash** my hair **every single day**, that's good right?

- an expensive hairdresser is a waste of money, right? Cutting is cutting and coloring is coloring?

- a 2 euro/dollar shampoo has the same effect than the one I buy for 30 euro/dollar at the pharmacy of hair salon.

When you pay attention to your diet and your hair growth, you will give it the power to support its growth from the inside out. Of course this can all go to waste if you don't treat your hair optimally on the outside.

If you want beautiful hair, you must be willing to dedicate the time for appropriate treatment. Treat your hair gently, with the right products and in the right way. Your hair is a part of your personality, of your look and it is being assessed by others when they see you for the first time.

Self-care does not equal vanity, it's a form of respect and love for your body.

A well-groomed and healthy head of hair gives you more self-confidence and shows the outside world that you deserve a place in it. This does not necessarily mean that you have to style your hair everyday. If you feel like it, great! But I love natural and I like to let my natural hair be like it is, that way I feel most comfortable about myself. But treating it well is something I will never skip.

In this chapter I share my tips and tricks for optimal hair care. I also give some product information to help you make a choice in the overwhelming selection of products on the market. My personal preference goes out to all-natural products, but for people who like to super style their hair, I will also list some brands that are not completely natural, but who process natural ingredients in an optimal way and have already reduced the number of hazardous substances, and from which I know that they are constantly looking for better and healthier formulas.

To obtain certain hairstyles, some additions to the formula are still necessary because there are no natural alternatives that provide the same professional effect, for example in hairspray to fix your hair or some smoothing products. However, I motivate those brands to never stop searching for healthier and environmentally safer solutions with the same professional results.

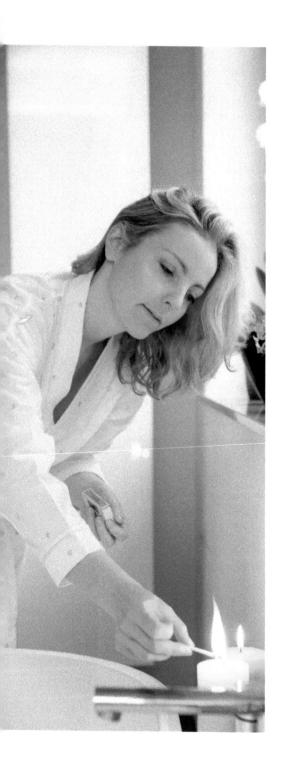

RESPECTING MOTHER NATURE

Why are we so obsessed with the style of our hair? Someone with curls wants to have straight hair and someone with straight hair, wants more curls. By frequently and aggressively trying to achieve a hairstyle that is not in your nature, you will destroy your hair. Give your natural look the opportunity to show itself and give your hair some rest.

Make the most of your personal, natural style. A good hairdresser knows how to advise you. If you have curls, make them even more fantastic so that nobody can resist them. If you have straight hair, a good hairdresser can make all the difference by giving you a good haircut or the right styling tips. A good cut if done well by a professional, will stay in shape for much longer. A skilled hairdresser will always make time for you, listens to your wishes and is an essential part in caring for your beautiful hair.

GET A REGULAR CUT!

Even if you want to grow out super long hair, it is important to get it cut once in a while. Every two months really is a must. This way the ends of the hair will be healthy, your hair will look better and it will fall into place perfectly. Be patient when growing your hair, rushing things is, as always in life, not a good thing.

Don't be frugal when choosing your hair salon. I have learned that a cheap haircut will often turn out to be more expensive in the end. A more expensive haircut at a high-quality hair salon, is really worth the money and your new style will last longer. Your hair 'falls' better after a visit to a good hairdresser who works with your hair, and not towards a hairstyle that isn't in your nature.

TIP

A bad hair day can be fixed by putting your hair up or by making a ponytail. When you choose to make a bun, it is best not to use too many metal hairpins. Choose a hair clip instead, that can hold your hair together, but doesn't break it. If you make a ponytail then choose a rubber band, covered with fabric and without any metal parts. The brands Babyliss, Invisibobble and Elle have fun and good pins and bands for every style.

Don't pull your ponytail or knot too hard, because this puts too much strain on the hair. This can result in a headache and if you do it every day, even in hairloss.

If I want to

off the front

change my

knock a story

page, I just

hairstyle.

HILLARY RODHAM CLINTON

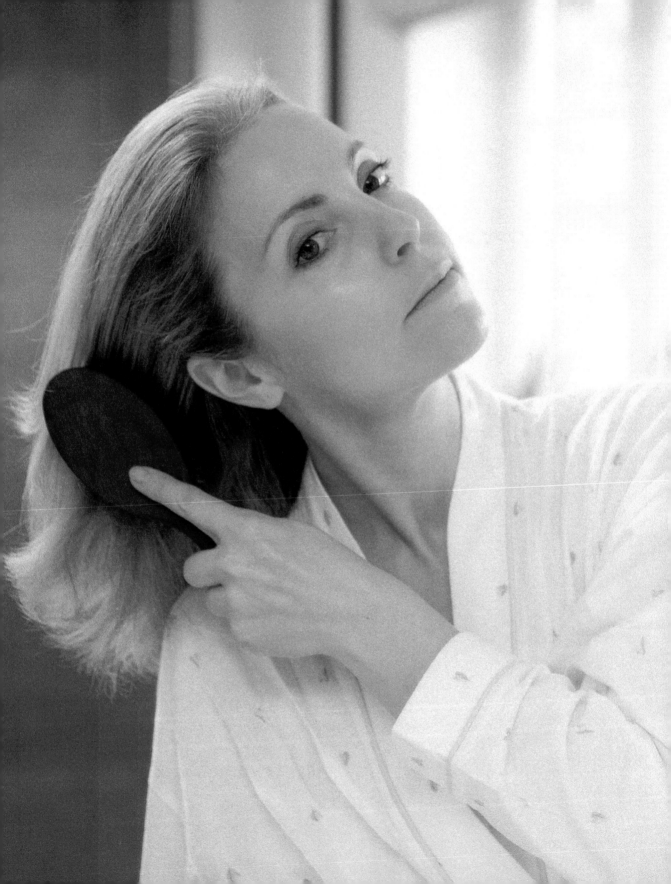

THE PERFECT WASH

Washing your hair well is a must for a fresh hairdo and makes your hair ready for the caring treatment that comes after it. During my small talk at the hairdressers, I have learned that many people do not wash thoroughly enough. This results in residue build-up from shampoo and styling products, which obstructs effectively washing away dead skin cells and dirt (dust, pollution...) from hair and scalp.

- **Before taking a shower**, start with **brushing** your hair to remove any knots. This limits the need to brush or comb when your hair is **wet**. For starters, make your hair soaking wet with **lukewarm** water.

- Apply a small **quantity of shampoo**, massage into the scalp and **rinse out**.

- **Repeat** with another small quantity of shampoo and wash your hair again, but this time more thoroughly.

- Use your fingertips to massage the shampoo in and don't scratch your scalp with your nails.

- **Rinse** the hair **very carefully** so that it's ready for a nourishing treatment.

Choose the right shampoo for your hair type. Get advice from a good hairdresser. It really makes a difference what brand and type you choose. Also in this case, cheap is more expensive in the end. If you use a good and more expensive brand, you need less shampoo and get better results.

TIP

Shampoo doesn't need to foam excessively. The foaming effect doesn't have anything to do with the cleansing or nourishing power. The foam, in most products, is created by adding sulphates that carry the name of 'sodium lauryl/laureth sulfate' (SLS). The higher it is listed on the label of the bottle, the more of the substance is in it. It is better to choose an alternative like 'sodium lauryoll sarcosinate', 'disodium cocoyl glutamate', 'sodium cocoyl glutamate' or 'disodium coco-glucoside citrate'.

Recommended brands:
Moroccanoil, Shu Uemura, Maria Nila, Aveda, Phyto, René Furterer, Rahua, Weleda, Madara, Caudalie

DELICIOUSLY FRESH

Cold showers and swimming in cold water is very healthy and invigorating. I love it! After washing and nourishing your hair, finish with a splash of cold water. It increases blood circulation, closes the pores and is good for your hair. You will probably need some time to get used to it, but after a while it becomes a (healthy) addiction.

A cold shower is also good for the immune system and there are many studies that show that an ice-cold bath is a particularly strong remedy for colds and helps restore muscle stiffness after exercise.

SKIP A HAIR WASH!

Not washing your hair every day, is one of the things that I and other hair lovers have found to be really beneficial for your hair. The sebaceous glands around the hair follicles produce a natural conditioner (sebum) that nourishes your hair perfectly. If you wash too often, that precious natural product will be washed out as well.

The more you wash, the greasier your hair becomes in the long run, creating a situation where you have to wash your hair more often. I myself wash my hair only every three to four days and sometimes I wait even longer. I take time to pamper my hair on an everyday basis with a good brushing ritual (see below) to distribute sebum on the hair strands.

If the hair on the crown of my head starts to look greasy, I will use a good quality dry shampoo (e.g. *Klorane* or *Moroccanoil*) or some natural talc powder to freshen up. When using dry shampoo the message is: less is more! If you use a dry shampoo in a vaporizer, spray it very gently targeting the spots you want to refresh.

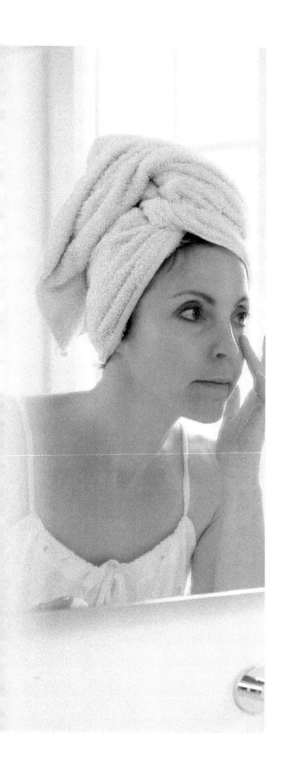

Massage it in like a shampoo and leave it in for two minutes before brushing your hair. Nowadays there are dry shampoos that are adjusted to the color of your hair. This way you won't have a 'white' effect (check the brands listed above).

When you're using natural talc (I often use *Dr. Hauschka* body powder, it smells delicious), apply a small quantity onto your hands, rub it between the palms of your hands and rub it onto the greasy spots. After two minutes you can brush out any excess powder. This natural talc is also my favourite natural deodorant and foot powder.

Dry shampoo is a real timesaver, your hair will smell deliciously fresh, you will get more volume and it all goes super speedily! I always have a bottle in my gym bag and in the glove compartment of my car.

After shampoo comes care. A good shampooing always has to be finished off with appropriate care. I deliberately choose a conditioner of a good brand, because you only need a small amount and the result is top-notch. Massage the conditioner in with your hands and fingers. Follow the directions carefully, because sometimes the manufacturer advises not to go all the way up to the scalp. Preferably use your fingers to comb through your hair until most knots are gone.

When you have more knots, you can use a wooden comb. Give your conditioner sufficient time to do its work. Remember to rinse thoroughly!

I also regularly use a hair mask: in the next chapter you can find some recipes that you can try at home, but obviously you can always opt for a ready-made hair mask to deeply nourish your hair. Good nourishment of the hair is a must, especially if you straighten or color your hair, or spend a lot of time in the sun or in the water.

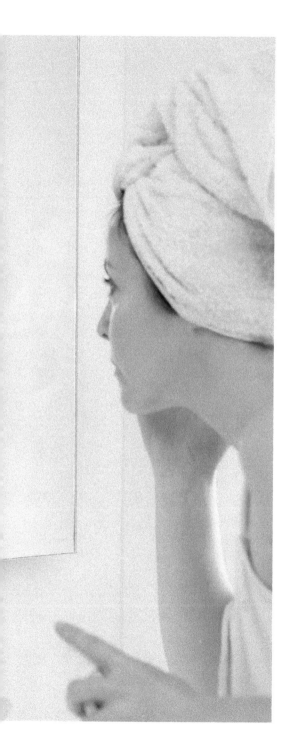

Take your time for deep care and in the mean time spoil yourself with a pedicure, manicure or facial mask. Recommended brands for conditioners and hair masks: *Moroccanoil, Aveda, René Furterer, Shu Uemura, Maria Nila, Phyto, Rahua, Madara, Weleda* and *Dr. Hauschka*.

LESS HEAT!

The heat from hairdryers and straighteners isn't good for your hair, no matter what brand they are from and especially when you use them in the wrong way and too often. Let your hair dry naturally for a change. If you want to use a curling iron, a straightener or if you want to go for a blow-dry, choose the very best equipment and protect your hair using a customized product (e.g. *Moroccanoil* or *Rahua*) that limits heat damage to a minimum.

I myself wrap my wet hair in a cotton towel for about five minutes to absorb most of the moisture. After that I let my hair air-dry and when it is dry I brush it for volume and shine with one of the brushes from my own brand. For more natural volume you can always try my method that I will discuss in another chapter: upside down!

DOS AND DON'TS FOR WET HAIR

Never rub your hair dry with a towel! Rubbing will destroy your hair. It's better to gently squeeze-dry your hair with a towel. Also avoid too much combing when your hair is wet, because when wet, it is very prone to breaking. I use a caring brush from my own range to go briefly through my towel dry hair to remove any knots. If you choose a good brand of hair products, then probably you won't need to untangle it.

I usually air-dry my hair. To add some bounce and volume to my hair without blow-drying, I let my hair dry completely and afterwards I apply a drop of nourishing oil. I then put my hair up, very loosely, with a big hair clip. When I remove this clip after about and hour, I just shake my hair loose and there you go, a naturally wavy hairdo.

MORE MASSAGE, PLEASE!

A body massage is such a bliss. But did you know that massaging your scalp is very good for your hair? It ensures improved blood circulation, making your scalp healthier and your hair grow better. Good hairdressers will give you a relaxing massage when applying a conditioner or hair mask, but you can always do it yourself when you are in the shower. Combined with the tips in the chapter 'Take You Time', this becomes extra powerful!

So get into the habit to massage your scalp while applying conditioner or a hair mask. Or use a wonderfully nourishing oil to give yourself a massage, or ask your loved one to do that for you. You can also stimulate your scalp by using a good quality brush, more about that below.

A HUNDRED BRUSH STROKES PER DAY

Our grandmothers already told us: a hundred brush strokes per day for beautiful hair. This is not a myth: I have discovered the truth behind it during the past two years in search for healthy hair. I really enjoy brushing my hair. I do it several times a day to provide my hair with some natural volume and shine. It's the last thing I do right before I go to bed, going through all that happened to then end my day.

By brushing with a good hairbrush, suitable for your hair type, you ensure that the natural sebum, your own conditioner, is spread all along the lengths of your hair and that it can nourish your hair. It is of great importance to invest in a good quality hairbrush because those are powerful enough to untangle your hair without damaging its fragile structure. A good hairbrush that respects the hair structure makes sure that the hair sheaths, which are imbricated to the outer layer of your hair, lie perfectly flat and as a result your hair is smooth and shiny. By brushing, your scalp enjoys a blissful micro massage which enhances the blood flow: oxygen and nutrients are more easily absorbed and healthy hair growth is promoted.

Finally, with a good hairbrush you remove dust, small particles from air pollution, pollen and dead hair. That way you make sure your hair can breathe freely and that it shines beautifully.

Grandma was right: a hundred brush strokes per day for beautiful hair.

DO YOU SUFFER FROM HAY FEVER?

Did you know that during the day your hair traps a lot of pollen? With a good brush it can be brushed out at night, so you won't be up all night sneezing.

Because I couldn't find the perfect brush for my hair and because I noticed that friends with more challenging hair types (like Afro-American hair, Afro hair, curly hair...) had a lot of difficulties to find a suitable brush, I wanted to find out what exactly makes a hairbrush a good one.

I became so passionate about it that I decided to develop my own hairbrush line named *Delphin & Emerence* that combines all the best features a brush can have. More than one and a half years of study and development in conjunction with Belgian craftsmanship that goes back more than eighty years in time, eventually led to a premium range of hairbrushes for all types of hair. More information can be found at www.delphinandemerence.com

Brushing is ideally performed with a natural bristle brush. The hair of the wild boar, called 'sanglier', is the best choice for that. Sometimes, depending on your hair type and when you have a lot of knots, a designated blend of natural hair mixed with a suitable synthetic hair type is a must.

A good hairbrush will cost more than a bad one. To make a good quality hairbrush, only the best materials are allowed to be used, which of course are more expensive. Quality is cheaper in the long run, because your brush will last longer, which is good for your wallet and the environment. A good hairbrush will not damage your hair so you will avoid costly repair operations that arise after using poor quality brushes (and you will especially avoid the frustration that your locks won't look good anymore).

We invest hundreds and sometimes thousands of euros/dollars on hair products, dietary supplements, cosmetic treatments and hairdressing sessions, but we forget that a good hairbrush is an essential part of our beauty routine and therefore a good investment in our appearance.

THE RIGHT BRUSHING TECHNIQUE:

I have already told my daughter a thousand times: "Do not chop your hair!" Always start brushing at the ends and work gently upwards to the scalp.

Softly brush out the knots and tangles, because wildly 'chopping' it with a brush will break the hair. I always start with a detangling brush from *Delphin & Emerence* and then finish off with a caring brush from the same line to make my hair smoother and shinier.

Especially avoid combing your hair with a metal or plastic comb, for these are too brutal for your hair. A quality wooden comb is a far better choice.

Because you chose to read this book, I offer a special discount code that you can use in the webshop from *Delphin & Emerence*.

DISCOUNT CODE

Go to **www.delphinandemerence.com** and use the following code when purchasing the product of your choice:

HAIRBOOK-2017

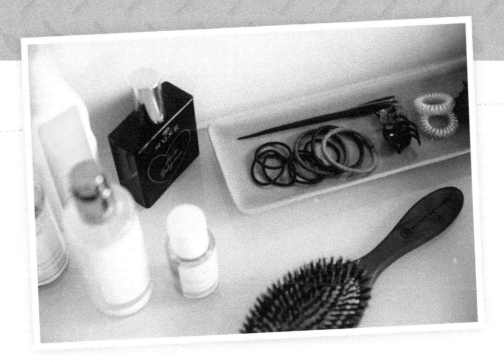

THE POWER OF OIL.

When I had very long hair in my teen years, I always used a nurturing oil. I rubbed my hair from scalp to tip with a vegetable oil, wove it into a loose braid and then always let it work its magic overnight or when studying for school. I used to apply, and still do, a very small amount of oil for daily care.

I made it my personal trademark because I perfumed the oil with natural essential oil of roses. Usually I use jojoba oil as it has a very fine structure which I then scent with some essential oil.

Nowadays I use a nice smell like a blend or a single oil from the brand *Young Living* (www.youngliving.com) or *Pranarom*. How much fragrance you add is personal and you should find the right amount that works for you. The reason why oil is so good for your hair and your skin is that natural oils are full of essential fatty acids and various nutrients. Even in a healthy diet good oil should not be missing.

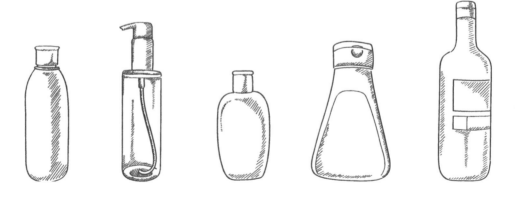

OIL AND TREATMENT

Good oils for an intensive hair treatment are: jojoba oil, argan oil (special smell but very good for hair and skin), almond oil, apricot kernel oil, avocado oil, olive oil, sesame oil, coconut oil and castor oil (ricinus oil). The last oil, castor oil, is a little different in texture and is in fact very thick and sticky. It is more difficult to apply, but it gives good results. For easier applying, you can mix castor oil with a finer type of oil.

Massage the oil for a deep nourishing treatment in both the scalp and the hair. Never spread it with your hairbrush, because your brush will end up very greasy. If you want, you can comb trough the oiled hair with a wooden comb. The best effect is achieved when you leave it in overnight. Always put a thick cotton bath towel on your pillow to protect it against stains. In the morning, wash your hair with a gentle shampoo and finish with a conditioner.

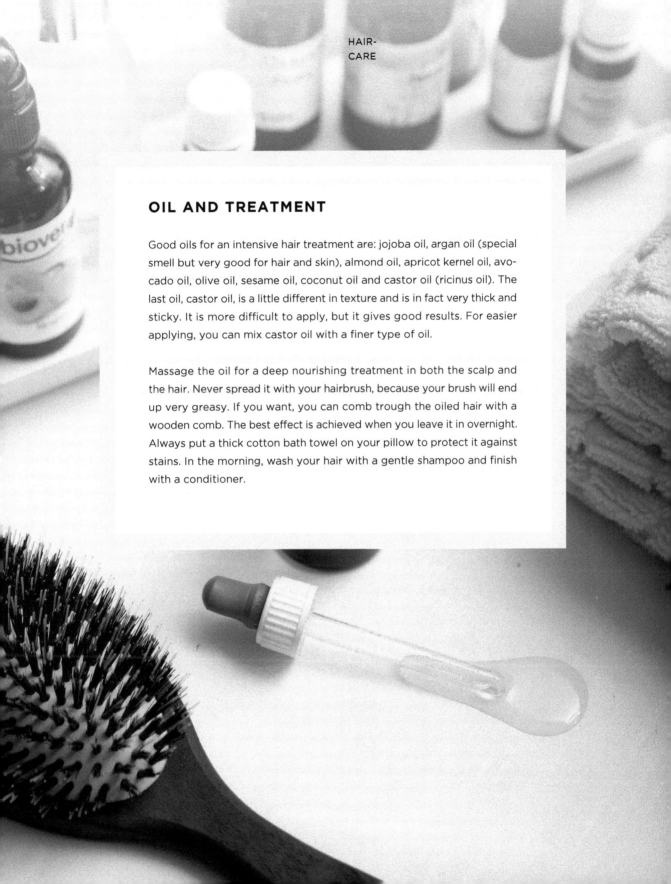

TIP FOR DAILY OIL CARE

Rub one to two drops of oil between your palms and massage it gently through the ends of your dry hair. Do not get too close to the scalp in order not to create greasy hair. However, with the last bits of oil left on my hands, I will sometimes run trough the hair on the crown, but only if I have just shampooed.

If I'm heat-styling my hair, I always apply a nourishing product such as oil, to protect the hair from heat damage. I then apply this when my hair is still moist.

The last couple of years I've also been using ready-made fine, natural oil mixes like the infamous oil of *Nuxe*, the caring oil '*Caudalie* Divine Oil' (smells delicious), 'Neem Hair Oil' (*Dr. Hauschka*), 'Moroccanoil Treatment', or 'Rahua Finishing Treatment' because, when used sparingly, they don't feel greasy and smell delicious.

When using one of the oil products, one or two sprays, one to two drops in your palms are enough to make your hair shine and to avoid frizziness. The delicious scent is a bonus and makes you irresistible.

STATIC ELECTRICITY

Everyone has experienced this: static electricity in your hair. It occurs more often during the cold winter months when the indoor air is very dry, and especially when you wear synthetic clothing, which generates more static electricity than natural fabrics such as wool, cotton and silk. Your hair may become more static by brushing, even with a good, natural hairbrush. This is totally natural. However it's certainly no reason to stop brushing! Brushing with a good quality hairbrush remains essential for proper hair care.

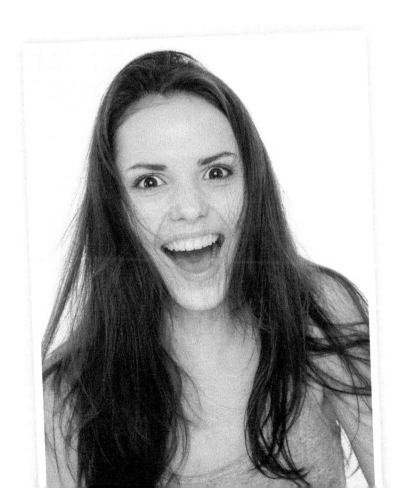

HERE YOU CAN FIND SOME TIPS TO HANDLE AND PREVENT THE SITUATION:

- Rub **a drop** of oil between your hands and go through your hair before you brush.

- Make sure to thoroughly nourish your hair with a **conditioner** and/or a **hair mask**.

- Only wear **cotton clothes while styling** your hair.

- If you dry your hair, opt for a **hairdryer** with **ionizing effect**.

- Ensure that **the air** in your home or office is not **too dry**. If necessary, use a **humidifier**

- **Avoid** friction with – particularly synthetic – **clothing such as sweaters and scarves** and avoid using plastic combs and brushes, they make the problem worse.

- **Rub** your hair with **wet hands**.

- Take a metal **coat hanger** and rub it over (not through) your hair. Metal is a conductive material and can thus discharge part of the electricity.

- Finally, even if your hair 'stands up' after brushing, do not panic. Give it some minutes and your hair will be perfectly relaxed again soon.

SEA, SUN AND HAIR!

How wonderful to enjoy the hot summer months or a sunny vacation amidst the bleak winter months! Swimming in the sea, in a fresh river or in that stunning infinity pool, not to forget the soothing warmth of the sun on your skin, delicious!

But we all know that the effects of sun, water, sea salt and chlorine are not exactly conducive to a beautiful skin and hair. Just as you protect your skin with a high protection sun cream to prevent sun damage and skin aging, you should also protect your hair appropriately. Oil is also a fantastic ally here.

Before you go to the beach, rub some natural oil, like we described in this chapter, into your hair. Now is the time to use quite a bit more than usual, because you are really going for protection. You can comb your oiled hair back for a wet look or you may, if you have long hair, put your hair up in a bun or make a beautiful braid.

A nice hat or a scarf is not only beautiful in summer, but also protects your hair and your scalp from UV radiation. And yes, your scalp can get sunburned! Protect your head and drink plenty of water so you don't have to cancel that fun cocktail party on the beach, because you are in bed suffering from a sunstroke!

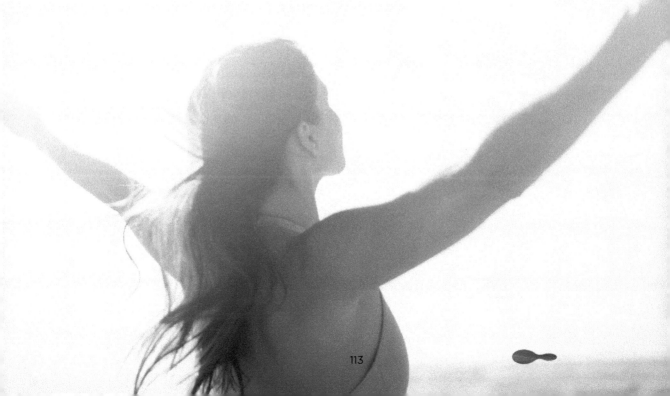

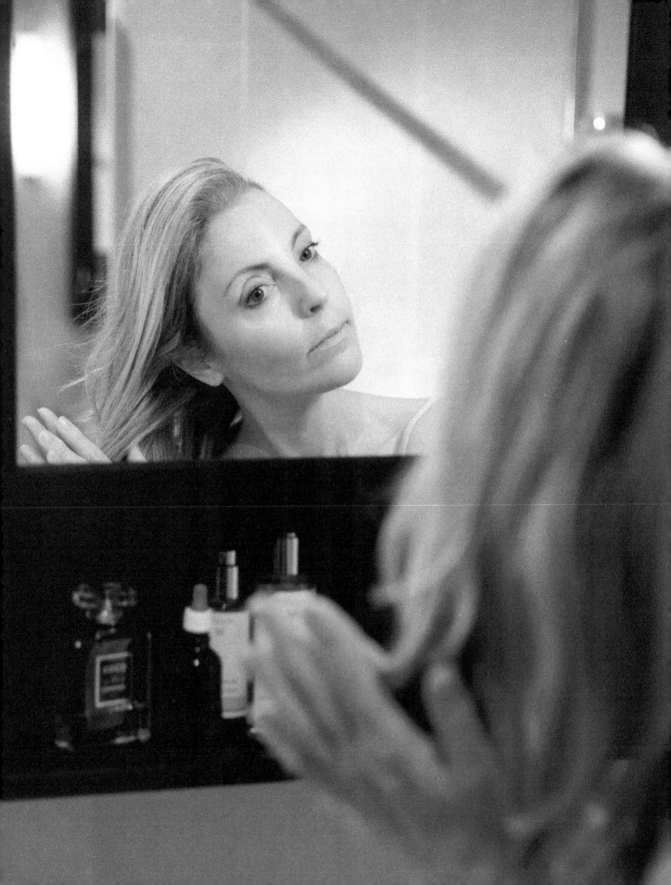

Today, there already are special haircare products on the market that contain a sunscreen. Ask advice from your stylist or pharmacist. After a day of sunbathing and splashing, wash your hair with a gentle nourishing shampoo and always use a good conditioner and regularly apply a nourishing hair mask.

Let it air-dry as much as possible to prevent additional heat damage from the hairdryer. There are a lot of nice products on the market to give your hair a beach look and to accentuate your natural curls and waves (e.g. *Moroccanoil*, *Rahua* and *Bumble and Bumble*).

SLEEPING BEAUTY

Sleep and adequate rest are essential for healthy hair and for your health. Sleep gives your body the rest it needs to recover after a busy day. When you sleep the production of growth hormone is being stimulated, promoting cell regeneration. This also benefits the cells in your hair.

Make sure you get a minimum of seven to eight hours of sleep. Young teenage girls need even more sleep to optimally develop their bodies (and their beautiful hair), they should go for nine to ten hours of sleep. Sleeping gives you a fresh glow, no concealer or blush is needed. It's much more effective than that foundation cream that young girls are applying way too early.

Everything you do, you'll do better
with a good night's sleep.

ARIANNA HUFFINGTON, AUTHOR OF THE SLEEP REVOLUTION:
TRANSFORMING YOUR LIFE, ONE NIGHT AT A TIME

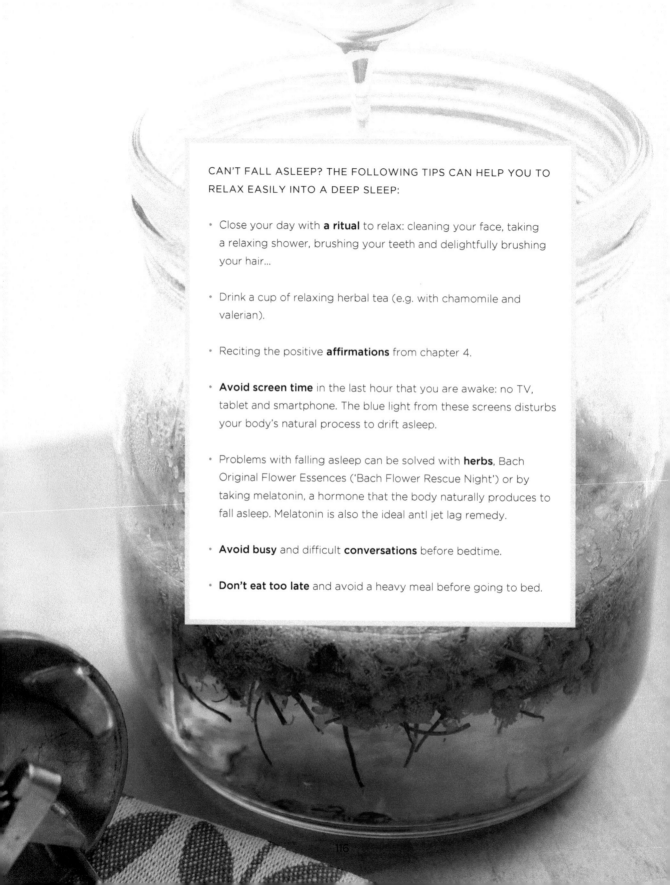

CAN'T FALL ASLEEP? THE FOLLOWING TIPS CAN HELP YOU TO RELAX EASILY INTO A DEEP SLEEP:

- Close your day with **a ritual** to relax: cleaning your face, taking a relaxing shower, brushing your teeth and delightfully brushing your hair...

- Drink a cup of relaxing herbal tea (e.g. with chamomile and valerian).

- Reciting the positive **affirmations** from chapter 4.

- **Avoid screen time** in the last hour that you are awake: no TV, tablet and smartphone. The blue light from these screens disturbs your body's natural process to drift asleep.

- Problems with falling asleep can be solved with **herbs**, Bach Original Flower Essences ('Bach Flower Rescue Night') or by taking melatonin, a hormone that the body naturally produces to fall asleep. Melatonin is also the ideal antl jet lag remedy.

- **Avoid busy** and difficult **conversations** before bedtime.

- **Don't eat too late** and avoid a heavy meal before going to bed.

When you sleep on a silk pillowcase you won't only dream very well, but it is also much better for your skin and hair. Your hair is less frizzy when waking up, because there is less friction, and you wake up without 'sleep wrinkles'. And did you know that you should regularly wash your pillowcase? At least once a week is the message, but I do it often two times a week and always have some spare pillowcases ready.

Pillowcases get greasy and dirty by using facial products for night care, hand cream and leftover dirt in your skin and hair. If your pillowcase is not clean, you will promote greasy hair and pimples.

HELP, I'VE GOT DANDRUFF!

Dandruff and flakes are names for an annoying hair condition. However, it has nothing to do with a lack of hygiene and it is not contagious. On the contrary, too much washing or an overuse of (wrong) hair products that irritate the scalp can even stimulate the problem. Dandruff and flaking can be the result of harsh hair treatments, caused by an inflammatory reaction in the scalp or because of certain yeasts such as *malassezia* or *pityrosporum*.

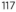

WHAT TO DO ABOUT IT.

There are many medicinal shampoos on the market to help you fix this problem. However, not all the ingredients in these products are natural and they do not always give a lasting solution after you stop treatment, and some of their ingredients can even make your hair very dry.

You can also find products (e.g. *René Furterer*) based on essential oils, in which especially tea tree oil (*melaleuca alternifolia*) plays an important role. In a later chapter I will give you a recipe, to create a treatment yourself.

If the problem persists, if you get small and painful lesions or if you get dry, flaky spots on other parts of your body, I recommend you consult a dermatologist. He or she has the best judgement whether your problem might be related to a contact allergy or psoriasis.

SPECIAL TIPS FOR FRIZZY HAIR AND AFRO-STYLE HAIR

To all those lovely people with frizzy, African-American or Afro hair: you were given such a beautiful gift from Mother Nature. It is important that you take good care of this precious gift. You have a very fragile hair structure and appropriate care is necessary. During the months I was doing research for my hairbrush line, I had the pleasure to meet a lot of people blessed with this fabulous hair structure, and found out that they were combing their precious hair with plastic and metal combs, severely damaging their hair.

Many treatments to straighten the hair and the use of hair extensions, in order to look like someone else, in the long run destroy and break your hair. This results in the fact that your hair gets so damaged that if you want long hair, you are 'forced' to opt for extensions.

I'm not an expert by experience with my fine, blonde hair, but during the many test sessions for *Delphin & Emerence*, I have encountered so many times that this type of hair needs extra special care and attention. When I took a closer look at the hair of the women in my test panels, a lot of them suffered from irritated, dry and flaky scalp due to many aggressive treatments, combing with plastic and metal combs and too little attention to the care of the scalp.

First and foremost, it is important that you start brushing with a good hairbrush specifically designed for your hair, so you can brush, without damaging your hair. Brushing gently through your frizzy, curly hair makes sure that natural sebum, which is present on your scalp, can be spread over the full length of your hair. As an addition, treatments using natural, nourishing oils help to heal your hair to deeply nourish and give the hair what it needs to shine.

This particular hair structure tolerates more rich oils such as coconut oil (choose organic) and castor oil, but also other oils that I describe in this chapter are excellent. Apply an oil treatment at least once a week and allow it to draw overnight. Do not forget your scalp, because it also deserves some extra care. Try to avoid the so-called 'relaxers' that make your hair smooth and straight, and avoid overexposure to the heat from hairdryers and straighteners. Too much tight braiding and hair extensions aren't good in the long term either. Let your hair hang loose more often. In other words: be inspired by the many men and women who are proud to make their own natural style, their natural hair texture, their pride and glory. Do not try to be someone else and love yourself.

It wasn't until I fell in love with Lisa - fell in love with my coffee-coloured skin, my full lips, my round hips and frizzy, black hair - that the rest of the world was capable of falling in love with me.

LISA NICHOLS IN THE MOVIE AND BOOK 'THE SECRET' BY RHONDA BYRNE.

COLOR ME BEAUTIFUL

Nowadays more than seventy percent of all women color their hair. It's one of the reasons why you can't find hair color on your passport anymore. Another shade in your hair that underlines your personality, can give a real boost to your mood. This book is all about how to obtain and maintain healthy and glossy hair, therefore the information I provide on coloring is not a how-to manual. However, I do give some guidance, some tips to color gently and to keep your hair healthy and beautiful during the process.

A permanent hair color, the kind that does not wash out after a few washes, colors your hair in-depth. The components in hair dye open up the sheaths of your hair, so that the color pigments can penetrate deeply into the hair cortex. Afterwards, the color in the hair will be fixated using a chemical component, like ammonia. It is of great importance that the hair is well cared for after a coloring session. This ensures the hair sheaths to close nicely and makes the hair smooth and shiny. Coloring your hair too often is something I would advise against. You can certainly ask for professional advice from your hairdresser.

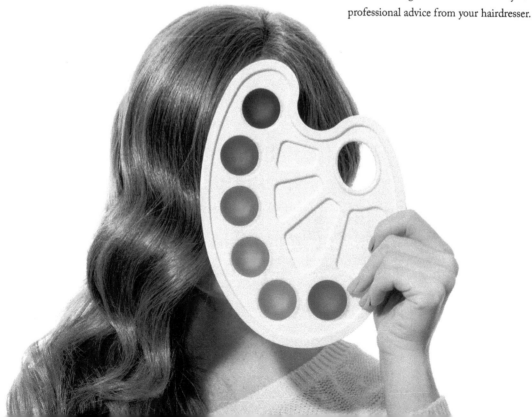

FINDING A HAIR COLOR THAT SUITS YOU

Choosing another hair color is very difficult, it's a specialist's job. A color needs to underline your personality and your beauty assets. Going for a good overall color match or just some highlights in combination with good professional advice can make the difference between a color that gives you a dull or artificial complexion, or one that suits you and makes your eyes sparkle and your skin look fresh.

A good hair colorist works with your natural features and tries to emphasize them. I often think about my father, who used to be a dentist. When bleaching the teeth of his patients, he also had the opinion that you can't stray too much away from your nature. This way the result wasn't only that his patients had clean and white teeth, but also teeth in a hue of white that looked natural. The same applies for your hair.

You can choose to color your hair at home, I do know a few women around me that do this with success, but I only let professionals do it, following the motto 'every man to his trade'.

I recently discovered that the Swedish brand *Maria Nila* developed a range of coloring shampoos, that are soft for your hair and give you a temporary color effect (nice to check how well a certain color suits you) or help you to maintain your colored hair fresh and lively between two color sessions. A great idea for your teenage girls to first try a crazy hair color in a safe way.

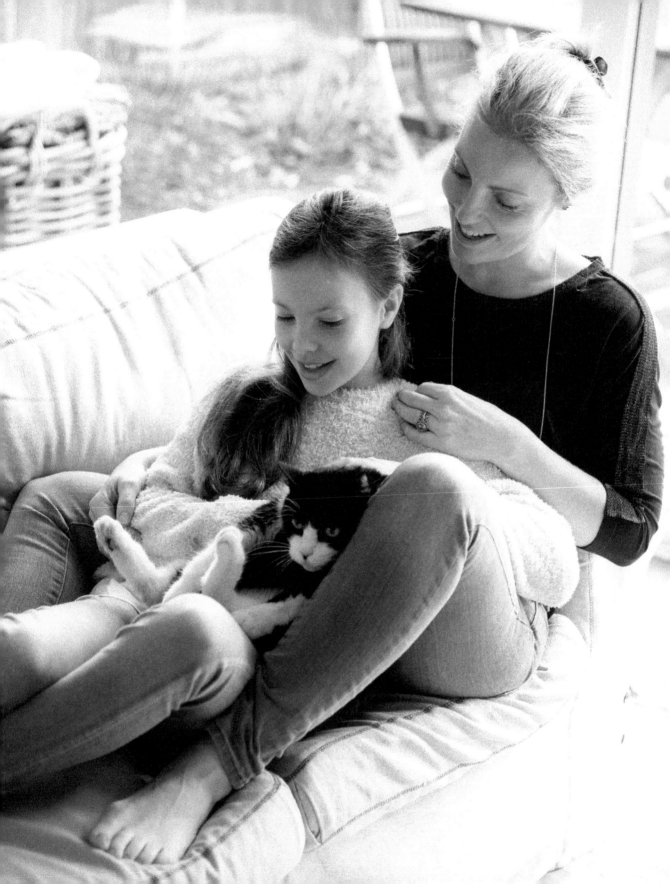

NATURAL BLONDE

- If you choose highlights like I did, then take good care of your hair. On the day **before** a **coloring**, treat it with some **natural oils**.

- Use an appropriate **shampoo** to **keep the color** of your healthy **blonde** looking nice. Your hairdresser can give you the advice you need.

- Don't forget, after swimming or when you're on holiday, to **protect** your hair from **the sun**, **chlorine** and **sea salt**. Before going for a swim, **rub your hair** with a **nourishing oil** and don't forget to wash it or at least cleanse it with pure water. A bathing cap or a hat can offer you the protection you need.

- By preference go for **natural highlight** products without any aggressive components. Since I made the switch to gentler coloring products, my hair structure has gotten remarkably better. Those products don't have such a strong smell and don't sting your skin when you are reading a magazine at the salon.

- If you like to maintain the **golden highlights** you got naturally from the summer months, you can choose to use the 'force' of nature. Extracts from chamomile will highlight your hair in a soft and gentle way. In the last chapter I will give you a recipe to use this herb.

NATURAL COLORING

In my teenage years I experimented with henna. Together with my girlfriends, we concocted our own brews to color each other's hair, ranging from brown to red or black. Sometimes it worked, other times it didn't. Since I am very fond of how I look – and I'm guessing that it is the case with you too – I decided not to color my hair myself anymore. I trust in the expertise and experience of my hairdresser.

Even though hair coloring manufacturers claim their products to be only based on herbs and to be organic, they always contain some chemical and hazardous components to fixa the color in your hair. The most hazardous component currently is PPD (para-phenylenediamine) or a related substance, PTD. This substance occurs with most brands, even so-called organic brands. It's a toxic substance that is hazardous for the environment and our health. The darker the color, the more of this substance it contains.

I'm not telling you to stop coloring your hair, I'm not stopping myself, but I thought it was important to tell you about this.

WHAT CAN YOU DO TO DECREASE THE IMPACT OF THESE SUB-
STANCES ON YOUR HAIR?

- Choose **lighter colors** (unless it doesn't suit you at all).

- **Don't color** your hair **too often**. The more time between two colorings, the better. This way you get less exposed to toxic substances during your life.

- **Take care** of your colored hair in a **proper way** (nourishment, less washing, protection), so your color stays nice longer. Ask a professional with expertise for advice.

- Refresh your hair color using a natural, non-permanent color shampoo, for example one from the brand Maria Nila.

- If you color your hair at home, carefully read the description on the package: **always wear gloves** and **don't leave** the color in **longer** than needed.

- Find a **formula without PPD**, although this doesn't work for everyone.

When pregnant, try to avoid coloring of the hair during the first trimester of your pregnancy. Avoid colorings that get in contact with your scalp, because your scalp will absorb this. Highlights are less dangerous, because they don't or hardly come in contact with the scalp. Ask a gynaecologist for advice when in doubt.

Often we are told that a certain product doesn't contain any ammonia and is therefore less hazardous. When the package tells you that its 'free of ammonia', the ammonia is often replaced by a substitute that also fixes the hair color in the hair and in many cases it is equally hazardous. Those substances are needed to give a good coverage and to make sure the color lasts longer. Natural colorings have the disadvantage that they wash out quicker.

My advice: get good and professional advice from your hairdresser + not too much + taking good care to limit the damage. Also, some natural extracts can evoke certain skin reactions and some henna colorings aren't as innocent as they look. Doing a small skin test is wise, also when working with natural coloring products.

Luckily there is an ongoing research for better, safer and more sustainable color-ings, so who knows, maybe someone will invent a 100% natural coloring product, which isn't hazardous, but keeps its color effect. In the meantime the brand *Maria Nila* is, in my opinion, the safest choice.

MY PERSONAL TOP THREE:

- less heat: use a hairdryer or straightener as little as possible

- invest in a good hairbrush and brush daily

- having a hairdresser with expertise is worth his or her weight in gold.

A good hairdresser is worth a million bucks.

Rapunzel,

let down your

I may climb

Rapunzel, hair, so that thy golden stair.

BROTHERS GRIMM

TAKE
YOU TIME

I love my Life!

22 december 2016

Dear Diary,

In this chapter I'm going to discuss the influence of stress, work-life balance and your mindset on the condition of your hair. In the previous chapters you learned how to take good care of your hair by eating the right nutrition for your body. Now I'm going more into detail about you as a person. How you feel, how you think en what goes on in your head has more impact on your health than you would think. For me, it was an important step in the process of healing my hair. In this chapter I will supply you with 'food for the soul'.

OUR BUSY LIFE

Stress, being busy and no time... have become the fashion words of our time and many of us choose to live by them every day. Back in the days, I used to have the feeling that I was 'being lived'. The days on the calendar flew by at lightning speed and I wasn't really present in the 'now'. I thought I could handle it all, that my battery could keep on running endlessly.

I was convinced that merely adjusting my nutrition and taking the right supplements in combination with a good hair ritual were going to fix my limp and brittle hair. Well, that turned out to be so wrong... According to the astrological zodiac, I am an Aries and they are the ones that sometimes need to bash their head against a wall to gain insight on their life. At the time of my health food restaurant, my customers funnily called me 'speedy' and my friends and family nicknamed me 'superwoman'.

I was always running around to serve everyone. My beautiful daughter Gina, the most beautiful gift ever, was born, in the middle of a super busy week at my restaurant. My gynaecologist told me – on a Tuesday morning – that my daughter could only be born safely trough a C-section because she was in breech position and... help... that the operation would be the next day. I had one day to get my business together for my pregnancy leave and ten days later I was back again in the kitchen, but this time with my baby. I committed to breastfeeding her for eight months. All this in combination with working six days out of seven. Sooner or later something had to give... The people around me noticed this faster than I did. One day I realized that I wasn't the same person anymore. My health was not in good shape, I struggled with food allergies, I was extremely agitated and exhausted. My hair reflected my mood and health situation and the word 'relaxation' was nowhere to found in my vocabulary.

It took me years before I really learned to relax and find peace, by meeting the right people and reading books and magazines that helped me gain insight, step by step, into my situation. It was exactly that moment of insight that made the change and made me rise again. In this chapter I happily share my experiences and techniques with you. But I recommend you find your own way, since I can only show you direction. My friends and coaches Saskia Winkler and Sally Gray will share their methods in this book that gave me the peace I needed so badly. I have to admit that I still have difficult moments where I'm about to lose it, but the techniques I learned can then take me back to a relaxed state, so I can completely recharge and ground myself to continue on my path.

I believe we women are all fantastic creatures and 'superwomen' that own a tremendous lot of power but we have to learn how to take better care of ourselves. 'Take You Time' has become my mantra, because if you don't take care of yourself, you can't take good care of others, your business and your projects. In that case you don't have the required power to make your dreams come true and help building a better world.

Take You Time is my mantra.

LIES HELSLOOT

SALLY GRAY ND
NATUROPATH, NUTRITIONIST AND HERBALIST:

I have seen countless clients over the years experience hair loss and hair quality issues in a variety of situations from chronic autoimmune disorders, gastrointestinal issues and endocrine disruption. In many cases the first thing that people notice is that their hair is not the same, but they don't take this as a 'warning sign' and their health continues to deteriorate before they take action. Once they are on a healing path, they often find their hair improve quite rapidly.

It is very important to address and treat underlying health problems. In the process of healing, not only nutrition and haircare were important but also dealing with stress was one of the primary factors to restore balance.

AWAY WITH STRESS... WHERE TO BEGIN?

To remove stress from your life, there is no such thing as a magic pill or a magical remedy that fits everyone. The relationship between stress and health is a complex matter.

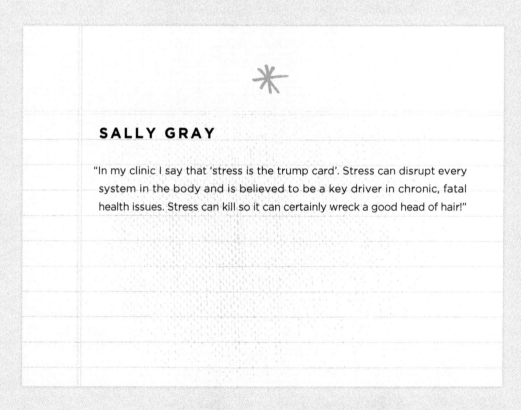

SALLY GRAY

"In my clinic I say that 'stress is the trump card'. Stress can disrupt every system in the body and is believed to be a key driver in chronic, fatal health issues. Stress can kill so it can certainly wreck a good head of hair!"

When you're under pressure and experiencing stress, your adrenals produce cortisol, which is dubbed as the stress hormone, and adrenalin. This mechanism prepares your body for a potential attack, in case you're being followed or attacked by a predator... Adrenalin makes your heart beat faster, raises your blood pressure and makes your body release the energy needed to attack. Cortisol also causes unnecessary body functions such as the digestive system, the reproductive system and growth processes to be disabled and it affects a number of processes that are responsible for the immune system. This whole process is useful when you are confronted with a certain dangerous situation and when you need to react fast and cold-blooded, but when the sources of stress consistently remain, as is often the case in today's busy world, then your body keeps on producing these hormones, causing it to become utterly exhausted.

The results are not to be underestimated: high blood pressure, heart disease, sleep problems, weight gain and hair loss. You can take all the supplements in the world and eat healthy, you can be taking all the right care of your hair, but if you don't bring more peace and calmness into your life, the problem will continue to simmer. Therefore, it is of great importance that you are also taking care of stress, if you want to be in good health and grow healthy hair.

We are all different and we live different lives. Therefore, it is important that everyone can find his or her own appropriate therapy. I have personally found – and I think many therapists will agree with me – that physical activity and some form of mindfulness therapy like yoga, learning proper breathing techniques and meditation can be powerful tools. In this chapter I will discuss some of those that played an important role in my own life and/or in the lives of others.

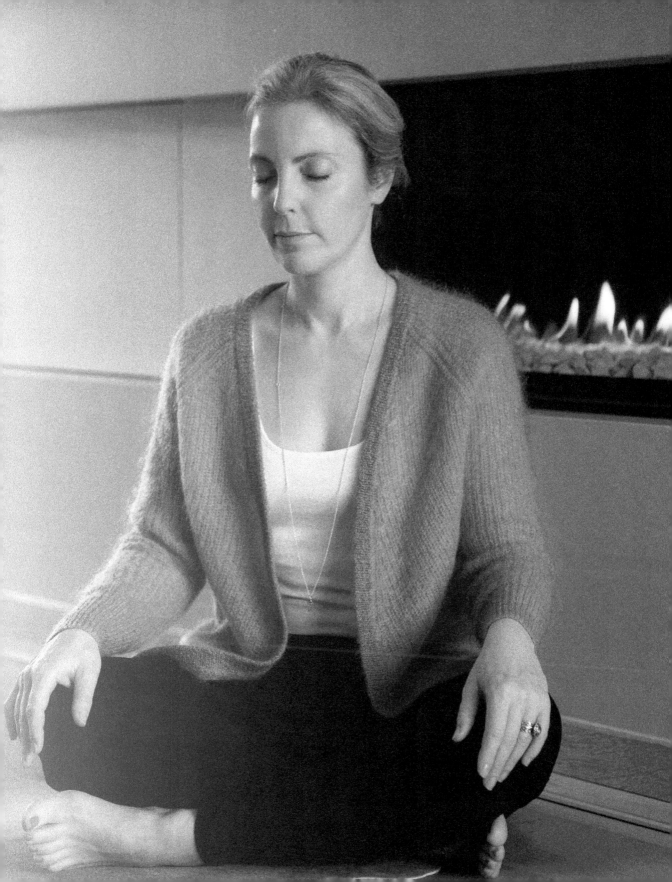

TAPPING OR EFT
(EMOTIONAL FREEDOM TECHNIQUE)

I got to know tapping for the first time during a seminar in the USA with success and life coach Jack Canfield. Thanks to my friend Sally Gray I refined this technique and I use it regularly as a relaxation technique. Even my daughter finds, in moments of restlessness, the necessary rest and relaxation through tapping. We enjoy going through this technique together.

WAT IS TAPPING?

SALLY GRAY ND EXPLAINS

EFT, or 'tapping' as it is more commonly known, is a powerful technique that anyone can do to relieve the body and mind of stress. Stress as we've discovered is such a powerful driver of dis-ease in the body and very often the reason behind hair changes or issues. Stress is a bigger part of life than ever which isn't great news for our health or hair. Finding effective and quick strategies that we can empower ourselves with can dissolve the stress we carry with us as well as create daily peace and calm.

Tapping refers to the action of literally tapping on acupressure points that are found on the meridian lines in the body as identified through Chinese medicine and the practice of acupuncture. Science now acknowledges the role that energy imbalance plays in creating disease. In fact, we are more energy than we are human cells so the world of energy and our emotions are where the secrets to health and perhaps life may be found!

Our energetic system is the realm of emotions, more specifically, stored negative emotions which act to disturb optimal functioning of our energetic system as well as our nervous system, the very system that informs our brain.

The practice of tapping works to release emotions and uncover the source of stress so that it can be released. We all carry stress in our energetic system and to relieve ourselves of this burden can only support our health and our hair.

The power of tapping lies in its simplicity. Firstly we become aware that we are feeling discomfort about an area of our lives. An example may be the emotions that come up when thinking about a stressful event from the past, or a traffic incident only yesterday. We then label the emotion that we can connect to the experience. This is a powerful practice in awareness just by itself. We then follow a set routine as follows allowing ourselves to consciously acknowledge the experience and emotions that we felt and at the same time accepting ourselves as worthy and lovable.

WHAT CAN TAPPING DO FOR YOUR HAIR?

We can use this powerful technique to also impact our hair. For more detailed information and a demonstration go to www.takeyoutime.com where I've created a video with the help of tapping expert Sally Gray ND to guide you through the steps to emotional freedom and empowerment.

SALLY GRAY ND EXPLAINS

• Identify the problem you want to focus on. (for example that your hair is not growing well) It can be general anxiety, or it can be a specific situation or issue which causes you to feel anxious.

• Consider the problem or situation. How do you feel about it right now? Rate the intensity level of your anxiety, with zero being the lowest level of anxiety and ten being the highest.

• Compose your set up statement. Your set up statement should acknowledge the problem you want to deal with, then follow it with an unconditional affirmation of yourself as a person.

• "Even though I feel this anxiety about my hair, I deeply and completely accept myself."

• Perform the set up: With four fingers on one hand, tap the 'Karate Chop point' on your other hand. The 'Karate Chop point' is on the outer edge of the hand, on the opposite side from the thumb. Repeat the set up statement three times aloud, while simultaneously tapping the 'Karate Chop point'. Now take a deep breath! Get ready to begin tapping!

Here are some tips to help you achieve the right technique:

- You should use a firm but gentle pressure, as if you were drumming on the side of your desk or testing a melon for ripeness.

- You can use all four fingers, or just the first two (the index and middle fingers). Four fingers are generally used on the top of the head, the collarbone, under the arm... wider areas. On sensitive areas, like around the eyes, you can use just two.

- Tap with your fingertips, not your fingernails. The sound will be round and mellow.

- The tapping order begins at the top and works down. You can end by returning to the top of the head, to complete the loop.

As you tap on each point, repeat a simple reminder phrase, such as "my anxiety" or "this fear" or "this despair"...

FOLLOW THE SEQUENCE OUTLINED IN THE
PICTURES OF ME WHERE WE SHOW THE
PULSE POINTS ON MY BODY.

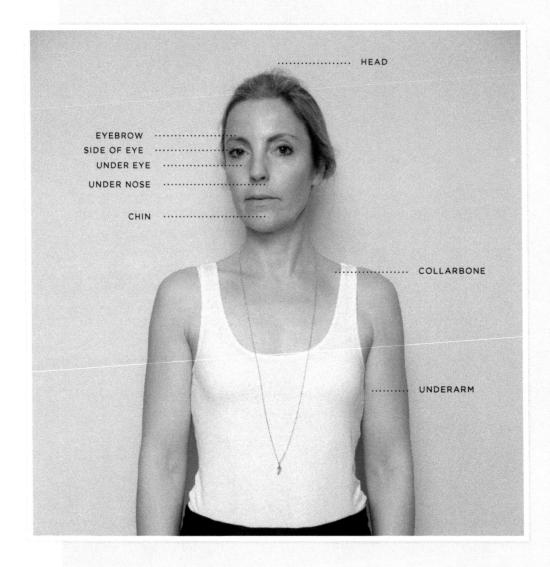

HEAD

EYEBROW
SIDE OF EYE
UNDER EYE
UNDER NOSE

CHIN

COLLARBONE

UNDERARM

HEAD (TH)
The crown, center and top of the head. Tap with all four fingers on both hands.

EYEBROW (EB)
The inner edges of the eyebrows, closest to the bridge of the nose. Use two fingers.

SIDE OF EYE (SE)
The hard area between the eye and the temple. Use two fingers. Feel out this area gently so you don't poke yourself in the eye!

UNDER EYE (UE)
The hard area under the eye, that merges with the cheekbone. Use two fingers, in line beneath the pupil.

UNDER NOSE (UN)
The point centred between the bottom of the nose and the upper lip. Use two fingers.

CHIN (CP)
This point is right beneath the previous one, and is centred between the bottom of the lower lip and the chin.

COLLARBONE (CB)
Tap just below the hard ridge of your collarbone with four fingers.

UNDERARM (UA)
On your side, about four inches beneath the armpit. Use four fingers.

HEAD (TH)
And back where you started, to complete the sequence.

Now take another deep breath!

NOW, TAP 5-7 TIMES EACH ON THE REMAI-
NING EIGHT POINTS IN THE FOLLOWING
SEQUENCE:

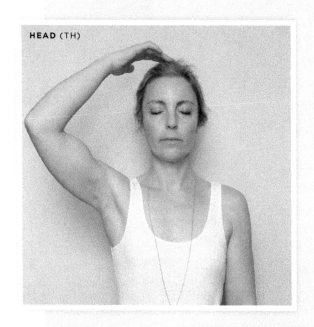

HEAD (TH)

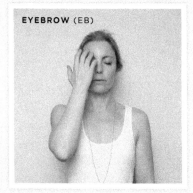

EYEBROW (EB)

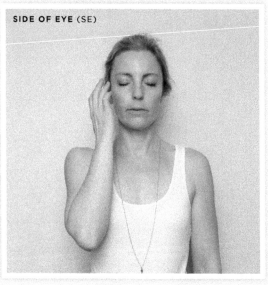

SIDE OF EYE (SE)

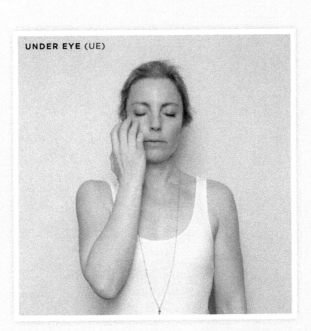

UNDER EYE (UE)

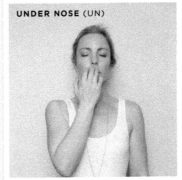

UNDER NOSE (UN)

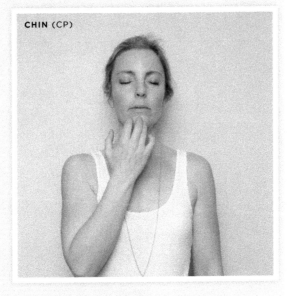

CHIN (CP)

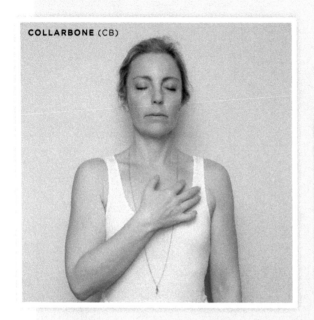

COLLARBONE (CB)

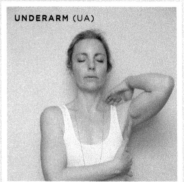

UNDERARM (UA)

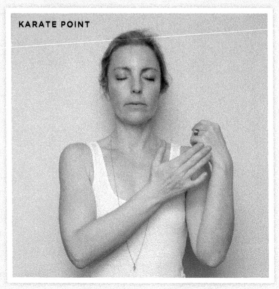

KARATE POINT

Now that you've completed the sequence, focus on your problem again. How intense is the anxiety now, in comparison to a few minutes ago? Give it a rating on the same number scale.

> If your anxiety is still higher than "2", you can do another round of tapping. Keep tapping until the anxiety is gone. You can change your set up statement to take into account your efforts to fix the problem, and your desire for continued progress.

> "Even though I have some remaining anxiety, I deeply and completely accept myself." "Even though I'm still a little worried about this interview, I deeply and completely accept myself." And so on.

> Now that you've focused on dispelling your immediate anxiety, you can work on installing some positive feelings instead.

Note: This approach is different from traditional 'positive thinking'. You're not being dishonest with yourself. You're not trying to obscure the stress and anxiety inside yourself with a veneer of insincere affirmations. Rather, you've confronted and dealt with the anxiety and negative feelings, offering deep and complete acceptance to both your feelings and yourself. Now, you're turning your thoughts and vibrations to the powerful and positive. That's what makes 'tapping' so much more effective than the 'positive thinking' techniques that many of you have likely already tried. It's not just a mental trick; instead, you're using these positive phrases and tapping to tune into the very real energy of positivity, affirmation, and joy that is implicit inside you. You're actually changing your body's energy into a more positive flow, a more positive vibration. Some help to get you started

This technique looks a little bit strange when you see it in writing and that's why a lesson from a tapping expert certainly is a good idea. If you would like to see an example of how to do this, I invite you to watch the video on www.takeyoutime.com. This video contains a tapping session that I, in collaboration with Sally Gray, put together. If you want to know more about this technique, then this is also a very useful source: the book Tapping into Ultimate Success: How to Overcome Any Obstacle and Skyrocket Your Results, Jack Canfield and Pamela Bruner, 2013.

RECOMMENDATIONS BY **SALLY GRAY**

- During treatment in my practice, in case of stress I often recommend a combination of the following supporting supplements in combination with a stress-reducing therapy:

- Collagen hydrolysate: a vital protein for the body that can be added to food and drinks

- Preparations with bitter herbs such as 'Swedish bitters' to support the digestive system, that is often out of balance because of stress, making sure nutrients are optimally being absorbed by the body

- Enzymes in support of the digestive system, both so-called digestive and systemic enzymes. A (orthomolecular) doctor can give you more information on this

- High-quality nutritional supplements, preferably organic as in the brand the Garden of Life (e.g. their multivitamins)

- Herbs that support the functioning of the adrenal glands such as Siberian ginseng, rhodiola, ashwagandha (e.g. in the supplement 'Metabolism T3T4' from Haylie Pomroy) and astralagus.

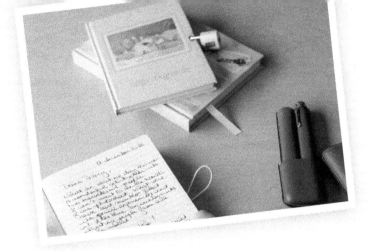

KEEPING A DIARY

As a child I always had one: a diary. The typical one with a dreamy photograph on the cover and a little lock with a key. I still have it, that first diary, and when I am feeling nostalgic I sometimes take a look at it. A diary is the perfect way to 'write off' my thoughts. It can help me place things in order, to vent some ideas and to get clarity in my mind. I don't do it everyday, there are times I write a lot, because I feel there is a need for it and there are times that I skip it. I do write a lot about my gratefulness for all the beautiful things in my life, being grateful that I'm healthy... and that I again have healthy, thick and shiny hair.

MEDITATION

There is a lot of talk about meditation, everyone has an opinion about it and knows 'the best technique'. I think that everyone needs to figure out for themselves which form of meditation is the best. To me, it can be as simple as closing my eyes and taking a deep breath. Or I will sit down under 'my oak tree' or underneath the willows in the meadow near my daily hiking route. Sitting there, I close my eyes, stretch my arms towards the sunrise or sunset, gratefully welcoming the feeling of the warm sunrays on my skin. Absolutely blissful... Also evening walks – especially around a full moon – give me that special feeling every single time. It makes me intensely happy and relaxed. No matter what happens in my life, the sun and the moon are always there and that is a soothing and calming feeling.

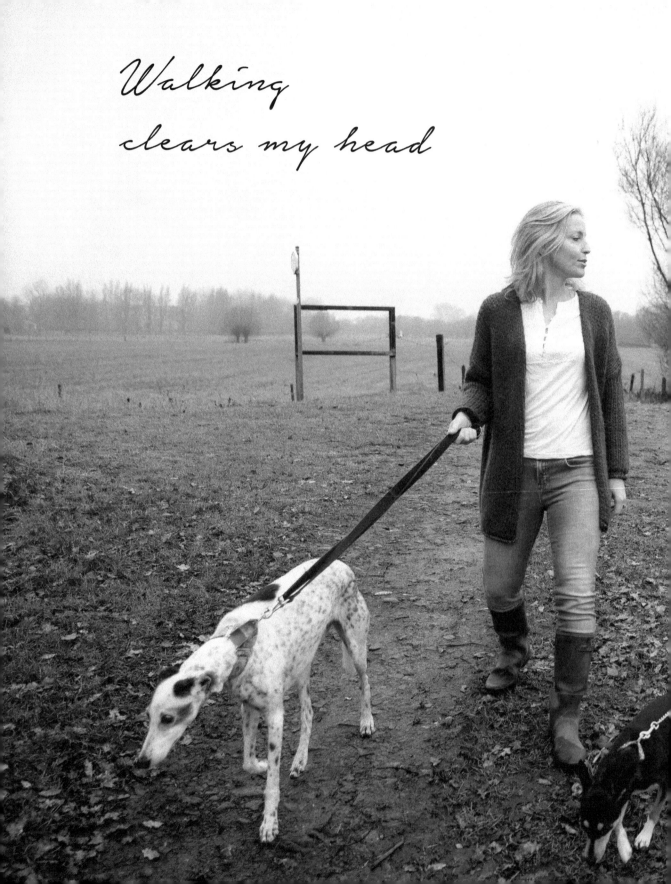

Walking
clears my head

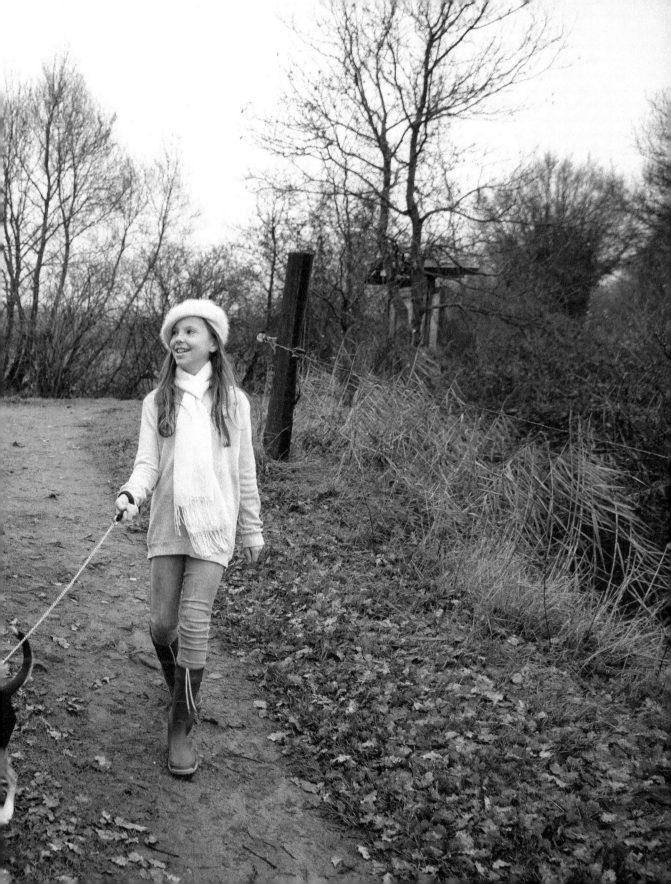

WALKING AND THE POWER OF A NATURAL ENVIRONMENT

Amid the craziness around triathlons and marathons, I remain a staunch supporter of walking. It is such a natural way to exercise and it is accessible to everyone. You really do not have to work up a sweat to get a good fitness level. Walking can be performed anywhere and, except for well-fitting shoes, you do not have to buy any special outfits.

Change your pace every now and then to raise your heart rate and try to find a route which offers more of a challenge, like one with a steep hill. Hiking has been a great help to me on days when I felt 'stuck' and worried. It clears my head, especially when I walk trough a natural environment with lots of green or when I can feel the sea breeze stroking my hair and see the waves rolling up the beach when walking near the sea.

Nature always calms me down and helps me put everything in perspective, it gives me inspiration and often makes me find the solution to the problems that are bothering me. Nature seems so simple, everything goes its own way, while we humans run around like a headless chicken, making life way too complicated.

Even if it's pouring rain, I'm in for a walk. The crashing rain that makes you soaking wet, is very relaxing and I often stretch my arms to the sky to be grateful for these refreshing drops. And afterwards, a hot shower warms your body and a cup of herbal tea tastes all the better.

I always have a pair of sneakers, rubber boots and a raincoat in my car. It often happens that, after a busy meeting, I make a quick detour to take a half-hour walk trough one of my favourite nature spots on my route. Don't be scared when you see someone in a skirt, stockings and rubber boots in the middle of the forest. There is a big chance that it's me or maybe, from now on, one of my dear readers?

YOGA

I am not really a yoga expert and never took any classes, although it's on my bucket list. In the library and on my coffee table I do keep a pile of magazines and books about yoga for inspiration. I often search videos on the internet from which I often pick a relaxing exercise. My yoga mat is always within reach for a quick relaxation exercise.

When I face one of life's moments when I think I'm going crazy, I will stand on my head. Crazy, right? Due to a car accident and a whiplash, I cannot perform a normal headstand, but instead I use a specially designed bench from FeetUp.

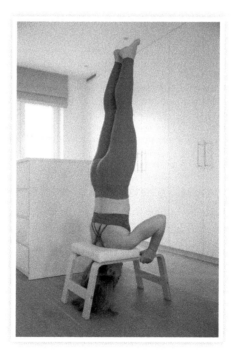

ON THE FEETUP WEBSHOP **WWW.FEETUP.BE** YOU GET A 5 EURO DISCOUNT,
USING THE FOLLOWING PROMOTIONAL CODE: **TAKEYOUTIME**

There are many different opinions about the beneficial impact of the headstand on your hair growth, but I am convinced that it promotes optimal blood circulation in my face and scalp, which can only help to get a healthy head of hair. After a headstand, I end up with a fresh, rosy glow – which is way better than from a jar – my back and shoulders are completely relaxed and ready for the rest of my day and a nice side effect is that I have warm feet because of improved circulation. It's just lovely to look at the world upside down.

MUSCLE-STRENGTHENING EXERCISES

A strong body also helps to grow a stronger mindset. As a young girl, you could almost daily find me in ballet class performing my favourite hobby: classical ballet. Nowadays I do muscle-strengthening exercises three times a week with my trainer Femke from *Lab'Eau* in an infrared cabin, alternating this with exercises at my house.

I always keep some weights near my television for a few quick arm exercises and a minute or more in plank position gives me that little bit of extra power to get me going. Just as my hair changed over the years, my body changed. With the correct exercises I was able to turn back the hands of time and I feel better than ever. I consider physical exercise as important as a business meeting. I committed to stick to my workout appointments, which rewarded me with good results both in a physical and mental way. The one who perseveres, wins!

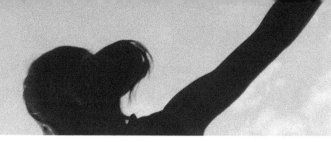

LET'S GO CRAZY!!

Why are we so serious? Do something crazy. Sing along with a happy song, do a funny dance, smile about your own bloopers and find a sense of humor in sticky situations. Stick out your tongue once in a while, it can be very freeing. How long ago have you done something that you really enjoy? There is nothing wrong taking care of yourself. You have so much more to offer when you are feeling happy and content.

HEY... CUP OF COFFEE?!

It sounds so simple and trivial, but taking time for a good cup of coffee (or tea) and a chat can help lower stress levels. The Swedes are very adept at enjoying coffee and even have a name for it: Fika. It is an essential part of their lifestyle. My friends Asa Katarina Odback and her son Emile Odback Nelson have written a book about it: *Fika Fix Your Life*.

Asa lived and worked most of her life in Sweden and ended up somewhere halfway in sunny Santa Barbara, California where one of her sons, Emile, grew up. Despite the pleasant climate, she felt that the American culture lacked the depth of a good conversation over a cup of coffee like she used to know in her home country. (Kind of funny knowing that the USA is often called 'the land of Starbucks'!) They wrote down the benefits of taking 'Fika-time' in a very nice book, a must-have on every coffee table. The meaning of Fika is about really making time for each other to get to a good conversation. You have to turn off your smartphone, so that you won't be disturbed and that the 'flow' of the conversation is not being interrupted. Swedish people do this several times a day, even at the office and they are convinced that this habit is promoting productivity in the office, because employees are more relaxed and happy.

Taking the time for a good conversation might be 'the' cure for the loneliness in our society and it works a lot better than the quick 'like' or 'comment' on your Facebook page. So, buy yourself a nice coffee mug with a cute saying and start chatting!

More fika time!

DELIGHTFUL BRUSHING!

Brushing with a good hairbrush is not only good for your hair – which I'll describe in the next section – but it can also be very relaxing. Especially if someone else is, lovingly, brushing your hair. It is the ideal relaxing moment for my daughter and me. I love to gently brush her beautiful long hair while watching a nice movie or one of our favourite episodes of *Gilmore Girls*. The perfect Valentine's Day present, although in my opinion you don't need to wait that long.

Brushing your hair can be part of your daily rituals. In the morning it will start you up for an energetic day and at night it's the perfect end of your day. While your are brushing, recite some positive affirmations and you can slide right under the sheets for a good night's sleep.

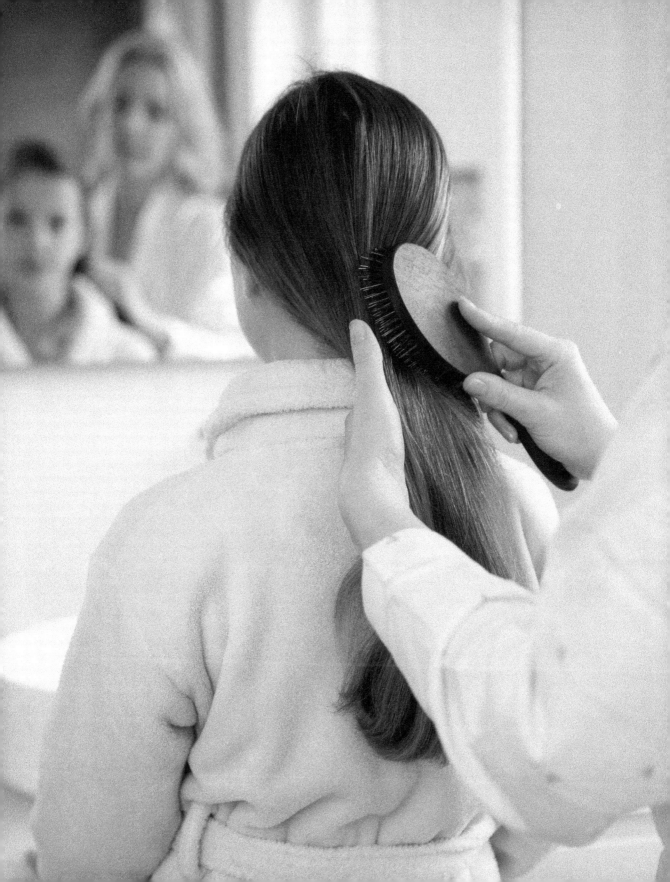

LEARN TO LOVE YOURSELF!

According to my good friend, coach, mentor and former CEO of Winkler Technik, Saskia Winkler, the body is a mirror of our soul. In an in-depth conversation with her in the context of this book, she shared her experiences with 'hair' in her practice.

"Especially our hair will show us how we feel deep inside and it shows us how we think about ourselves. There are countless examples of people who lose their hair. One of the worst cases I've encountered in my practice, were people pulling out their hair because they hated themselves, often not realizing why they were doing this.

Caring for your hair also requires caring for yourself and above all starting to love yourself again. Many women lose their hair after pregnancy. It is said that this is due to an imbalance in hormone levels, but I also see the deeper, more spiritual reason behind it.

Women often lose their hair during this period due to the transformative, immersive experience that the birth process brings along and often it is also due to a lack of support and understanding from the husband and family during this phase in their lives.

What happens is that, when you look at the connection between body and soul, the body and the soul seem to have decided to destroy the female beauty. In those women I then see hair loss on the crown of the head.

Also, people who have experienced a large dose of drama in their life, or experienced a traumatic event are often affected by hair loss. It is as if they literally don't want to be seen anymore. Again, the subconscious then makes sure that they really become invisible and unobtrusive.

The most common emotions that I see associated with hair loss, are fear and self-hatred. When people in my practice start solving their problems by recognizing shocking experiences, by forgiving themselves and by learning to love their own unique self and their body, I see their hair problems quickly improving. Even the structure of their hair is often totally different than before and it also grows faster.

I can't bring salvation to your reader's problems and fears by giving you a couple of sentences for this book, but from my experience as a coach, I can share some exercises and tips with your readers that can help them to grow healthy and luscious hair."

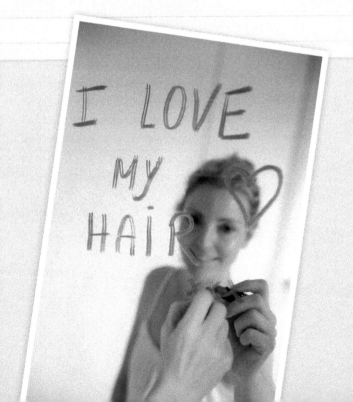

EXERCISES

The exercises that Saskia Winkler shared with me, will be described down below. I hope that they can help you. If you want to go deeper and get more personal coaching, you can get in touch with her through www.saskia-winkler.com

EXERCISE 1

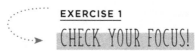

CHECK YOUR FOCUS!

When you are in your bathroom and look in the mirror, focus on the parts of your hair that you do love, not the ones you don't. Observe yourself without judging and focus in general on all the things you like about your body. In our society we are being urged on a daily basis, to look exactly at what we don't like about ourselves and to strive towards a photoshopped version of ourselves, which is far away from our true nature.

If you observe your hair and think you have too little hair, then, for example, you can focus on the color of your hair, that beautiful unique color that's only yours. Or maybe you have a special hair structure? And maybe you have more places with hair than without or with thinning hair? If your hair is too thin and fine, then perhaps it's very soft?

Run your hands and fingers through your hair in a loving way. Isn't that delightful? Make a list of what you like about your hair. And if you have no hair, make a list of what you do like and consider to be unique about yourself. Maybe then you will create more time for other things in life than to stand in the bathroom in front of the mirror? Maybe you're a stunner with that cute hat or scarf?

"It's just like when I have a pimple. I keep focussing on it the whole time, applying 101 ointments, using a camouflage stick to then come to the conclusion that in fact no one really noticed that I, in my opinion, have a gigantic pimple. It is better to focus on other assets and to shine, so put that smile on your face and let others see that."

Learn to love yourself.

THE POWER OF AFFIRMATIONS

Reciting, reading and writing affirmations is extremely powerful. For example, write on your mirror, 'I love my hair!' so you see it every morning and evening, when, for example, you are brushing your hair. Or make a nice note or Post-it with those words. If in the beginning you have difficulty saying the word 'love', then replace it with 'I think my hair is nice'.

Make sure you see this affirmation wherever you are taking care of your hair. Place it on the make-up mirror in your handbag, on a note above your bed, in your gym bag, on the dashboard in the car...

It is important that you do this every day for 21 days, making sure that you speak out loud and that you really do this with full dedication. Put your heart into what you say.

You can apply these affirmations anywhere. There is a nice postcard on my mirror that says: "Thank you God for making me fabulous!" When I feel a cold or flu coming up, I constantly tell myself: "I am fit and healthy, I feel fit as a fiddle!" The right mindset is so powerful that I made it a daily habit.

SOME IDEAS FOR AFFIRMATIONS THAT APPLY TO YOUR HAIR:

- I'm so proud of my fabulous hair.

- I am so glad that my hair grows so healthy and strong.

- I'm fine as I am, and others also think of me that way.

- I am blessed with my healthy head of hair!

- I have soft, shiny and strong hair.

- Every day is a good hair day!

- My hair is regrowing, thank you!

- I am happy and satisfied with my beautiful hair.

- I have incredible and amazing hair!

- Because of my beautiful hair, I'm irresistible.

- I love my beautiful and unique hair color.

- Nobody has such beautiful curls like I do.

- I love myself!

EXERCISE 3

STOP JUDGING!

There is no good or evil. Your hair is not bad. It's your hair. If you lose it, then the good thing is that your body wants to show you something. Something that can lead to a change process, if you decide to do something about it.

EXERCISE 4

IT STARTS WITH YOU: IT'S YOUR CHOICE!

There is a saying that regularly comes to my mind. Henry Ford once said: "Whether you think you can or you think you cannot; you're right." This can also apply to how you think about your health and your hair. You can either choose to constantly think, 'I hate my hair. My hair is ugly.' Or you can choose to be strong and to accept what is. Loving your hair starts with the acceptance of the situation you're in and with the situation you are aiming for in the future.

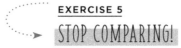

EXERCISE 5

STOP COMPARING!

I started to feel good in my life when I stopped comparing myself to others. Saskia Winkler helped me to further explore this habit. It all comes back again to the foundation, to you. Focus only on yourself. Do not compare yourself to others. You are unique, there is no other person like you. There is only one person with your name, your age, your thoughts, your voice and your character! No one can be like you, so please stop trying to be someone else and stop wishing you had the kind of hair that someone else might have.

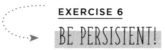

EXERCISE 6

BE PERSISTENT!

Making a change in how you think about yourself and your hair does not happen overnight. My dear friend Saskia gave me an example to illustrate this, especially because she knows I'm impatient by nature: "I remember a famous movie actor who was asked in an interview how it felt to suddenly, from one day to another, be successful. He replied that he did not know how many days and nights it had taken him to 'from one day to another' finally be famous and successful."

I learned from Saskia that my brain needed to be trained like you train your body in a fitness centre. Those who want a fit body must persevere and work out regularly to see results. It's the same with your brain: train it every day using the above steps and be persistent. I do recommend professional coaching when you find this difficult, because a good coach can help you keep your focus.

A women who

hair is about

her life.

cuts her

to change

COCO CHANEL

RECIPES

FOR
HEALTHY HAIR

Doesn't it feel good to make your own masks and hair treatments? As I told you before, when I was a child I lived with my parents in the countryside where my mother taught me how to make natural remedies for every kind of purpose. Besides the many herbal remedies for different ailments, my mother made all kinds of ointments and lotions for the treatment of wounds, pains and for taking care of our long hair.

For example, we didn't use lipstick for the care for our lips, but instead we got a little jar of lanolin to protect our lips and dry cheeks from the cold weather. Lanolin was a farmer's remedy and originates from the grease of sheep wool. It was a versatile remedy that didn't just nourish your skin, but also lubricated the zipper of your jacket when it got stuck!

All these recipes are engraved in my memory and give me a warm feeling when thinking of the many moments that I sat on the kitchen counter with my mother, drinking a cup of real broth and eating toast with marrowbone, while some kind of herbal treatment was boiling on the stove.

All these memories and tips that I gathered and tested, are written down right here in this chapter. I wish you a lot of fun preparing them and hope that it gives you my love and admiration for nature.

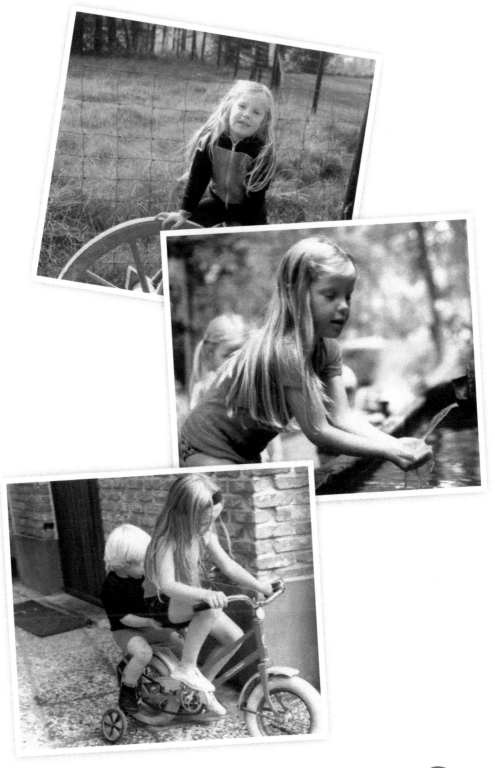

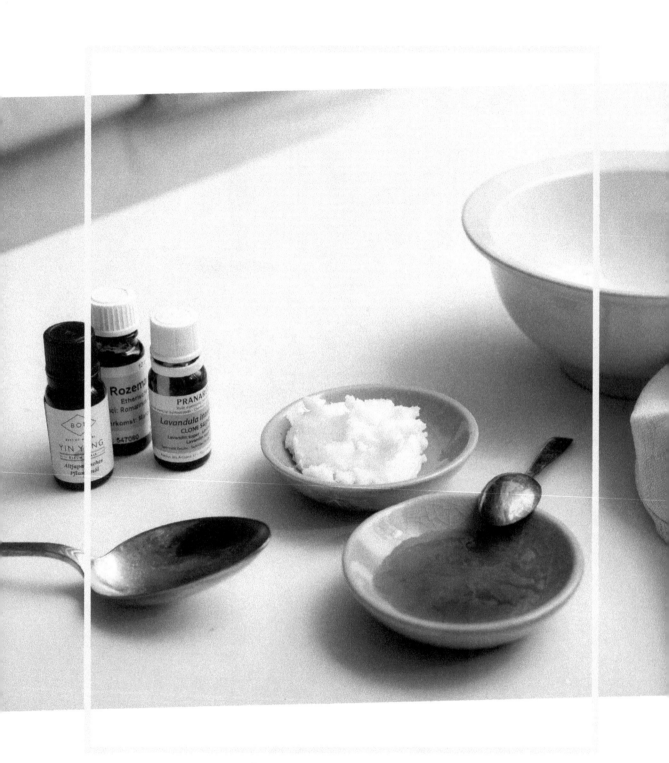

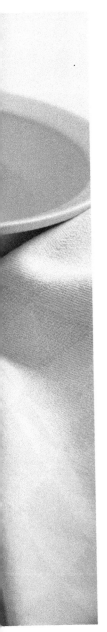

COCONUT-ALOË HAIR MASK

Coconut oil is commonly used for the care of hair and scalp in India and other parts of Asia and has, in recent years, become increasingly popular in both cosmetics and in the kitchen.

MIX

- 2 tablespoons of extra-virgin coconut oil (preferably from the health food store)

- 2 tablespoons aloe vera (also from the health food store)

- 2 drops each of the following essential oils: rosemary, peppermint, and lavender.

- Massage this fragant oil into your hair and scalp and then twist your hair in a towel. This is truly a blissful hair mask and thanks to the wonderful fragrances, a deliciously relaxing treat. Apply it weekly for optimal results..

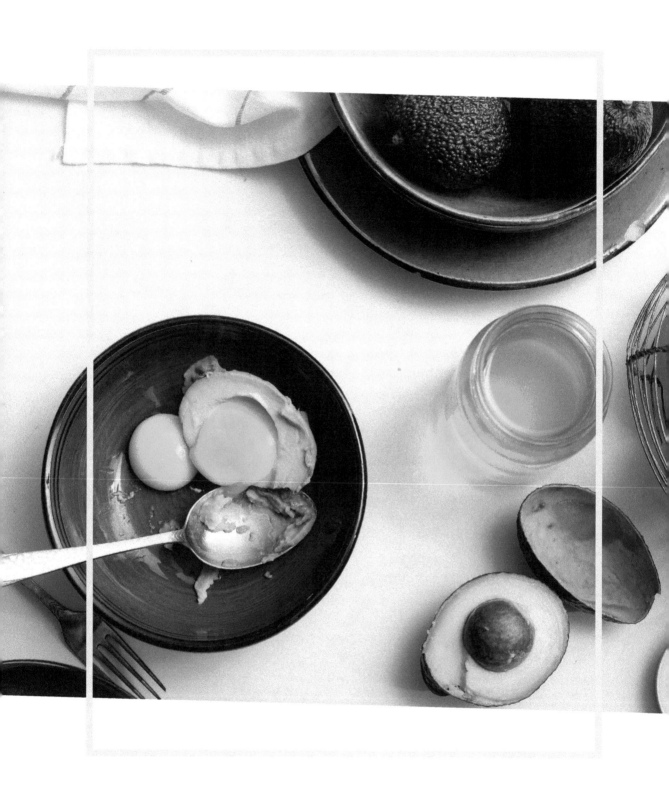

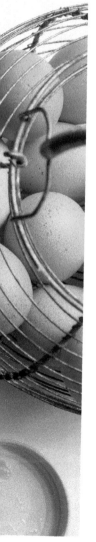

AVOCADO-EGG-HONEY MASK

This really is a deeply nourishing mask.

MIX

- To make the mask, mix two egg yolks, half of a ripe avocado and a spoon of organic, raw honey.

- Wash your hair and dry it gently with a towel. Apply the mask on your moist hair, wrap a towel around it and let the mask soak in for half an hour to an hour. Rinse thoroughly with lukewarm water (pay attention, hot water will turn the eggs into scrambled eggs).

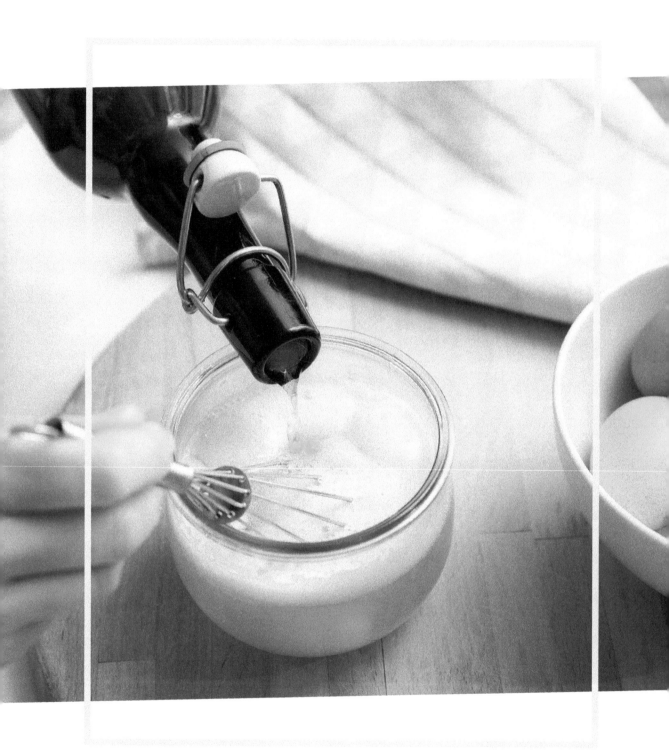

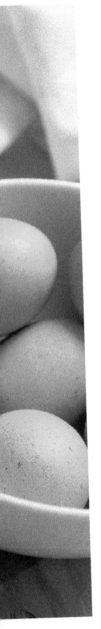

MORE VOLUME: THE BELGIAN WAY!

We Belgians are beer lovers and we are proud of the many delicious beers we brew on Belgian soil. But did you know that beer is also good for your hair? It's an amazing remedy to give your hair more volume and to make it stronger. It was a favourite treatment to do with friends when I was living in my college dorm room during my university days.

You can give this beer mask a try:

MIX

- 3 eggs

- 15 cl (5 fluid ounces) beer (you can enjoy drinking the rest of the bottle).

- Mix everything with a fork, a blender or a mixer. Apply the mixture to your hair and leave it in for half an hour, then rinse it thoroughly with lukewarm water (pay attention, hot water will turn the eggs into scrambled eggs).

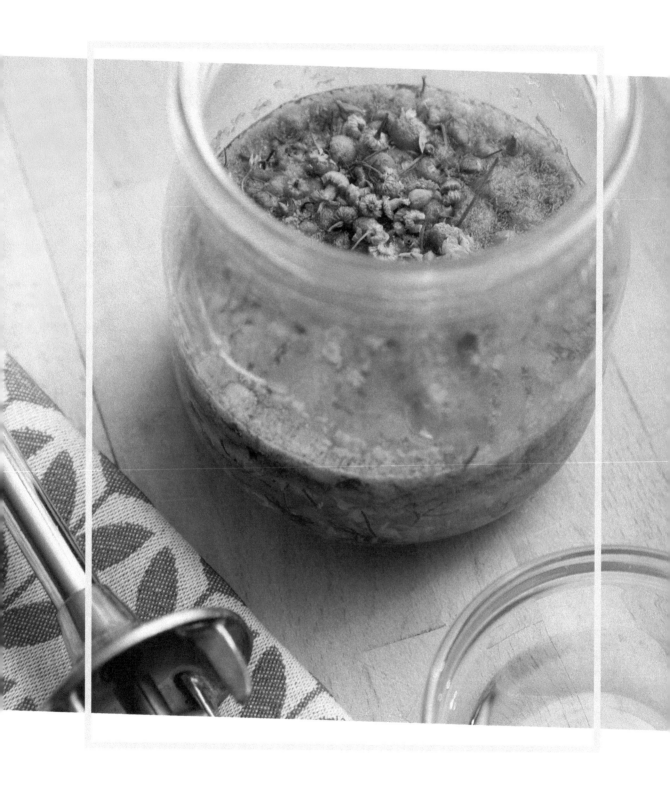

CHAMOMILE MASK FOR NATURAL HIGHLIGHTS

When I was little and living in the countryside, we always went to the fields with my mum to pick baskets full of chamomile flowers. Mama dried them in the sun or in the oven so we always had a good supply to use in tea, lotions and chamomile rinses to prolong the natural highlights of the summer months in our beautiful long hair.

At that time my mom made a strong decoction of these herbs which she then used to rinse our hair after washing, but over the years I started to use the herb in a different way, because I felt that it was more practical and powerful in a hair mask. But still, simply making a strong tea of fresh or dried chamomile flowers also works perfectly as a rinse. If you choose the rinse, then don't wash your hair afterwards so that the chamomile can work its enlightening magic and the delicious smell remains.

MIX

- About 20 grams (0.70 ounces) of dried chamomile flowers

- 150 ml (5 fluid ounces) of hot water

- 3 tablespoons of the oil of your choice (coconut, jojoba, apricot or olive oil).

METHOD

- Let the chamomile flowers steep for at least 30 minutes in hot water.

- Mix this mixture with the oil and mix it until it has become a smooth paste (I use a blender in a tall jar).

- Massage this mixture into your hair and wrap your head in cling film (easiest way) or a moist towel. Leave it in for an hour and then rinse out thoroughly.

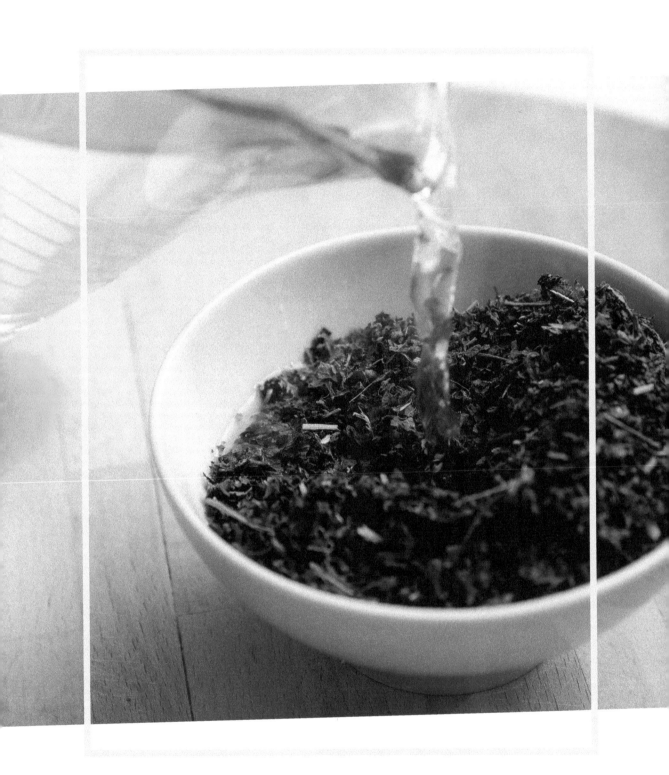

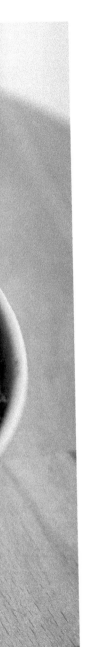

NETTLE WATER

Nettles do not only give you those itchy bumps, they can also be useful in the kitchen and in the bathroom. In the kitchen they can be used in soups, tea and pancakes and in the bathroom they make for a powerful strengthening hair rinse. You can also find over-the-counter hair products that have nettle in them.

To create a treatment, you can pick a dozen beautiful nettles, preferably in spring. Don't forget to wear gloves and protect the skin on your arms and legs!

METHOD

- Chop up the nettle into large pieces.

- Heat a pot filled with 1 liter (34 fluid ounces) of water until it boils.

- Add the nettles.

- Let it boil for 1 minute and turn off the heat.

- Let the mixture steep for another 10 minutes and let it cool down.

- You can use it to rinse your hair after you've washed it.

If you don't have fresh nettles, then make an infusion of dried nettles from the health food store.

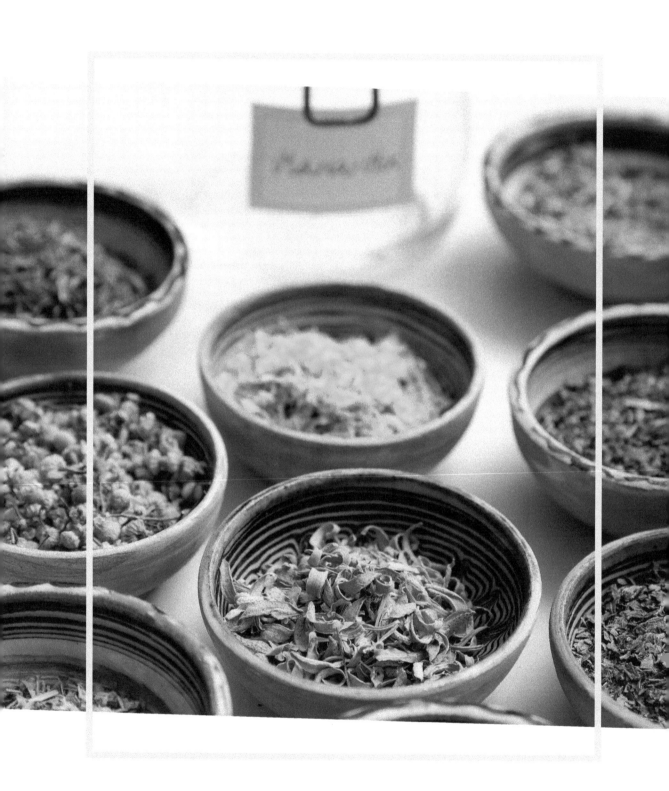

MAMA-MIX: RECIPE OF MY SPECIAL HERBAL TEA.

I once made this herbal tea myself with different herbs from the health food store. Many guinea pigs and I thought it was so good that I now have a batch in my cupboard all the time. I labelled the jar 'mama-mix' and ever since, it has become a household name. I do sometimes make other herbal variations by adding something else, but most of the time I stick to the herbs that are in the recipe below. This tea is not only good for your hair, but also for your general health and digestive system. Moreover, it is simply delicious with or without honey.

INGREDIENTS

Use a big bowl to mix the following herbs :

2 tablespoons lavender

6 tablespoons of chamomile flowers

6 tablespoons marigold

2 tablespoons blueberry leaves

2 tablespoons raspberry leaves

4 tablespoons orange blossom

2 tablespoons viola tricolor
   (sometimes called 'wild pansy')

4 tablespoons orange leaves

4 tablespoons of common (stinging) nettle

3 tablespoons of burdock

6 tablespoons of horsetail

3 tablespoons olive leaves.

- After mixing, put the herbs in a big glass jar with a lid. You can choose to use other ratios of herbs or leave out certain things. I do encourage you to make your own mix, but this one is simply very good and healthy!

- The advantage of this mix is that certain beneficial herbs, that some people might find not so tasty, are being blended into a mix that many will relish.

- Nowadays you can find dried herbs fairly easy online, but I usually buy them from a health food store like for example *Bio Shop, Origin'O, BIO-planet* or *Whole Foods Market*.

DIVINE OIL-TREATMENT

———

Create a mix with 4 tablespoons of one or more natural oils like jojoba oil, argan oil or castor (ricinus) oil... adding 3 drops each of the following essential oils: rosemary, peppermint and lavender.

Currently four tablespoons of oil are sufficient for my hair length, if you have longer hair it can be that you need more oil. Massage this mixture into the scalp and divide it over the lengths of the hair. Let it sit for as long as possible. I usually leave it on overnight, but sometimes I just leave it to do its work for about an hour while I am working on my computer.

Afterwards rinse out with a gentle shampoo.

TIP

If you often use oils in the bathroom, you can have trouble with clogged drainpipes. I made it a habit to regularly (twice a month) pour a bucket of very hot water and a handful of dissolved soda granules in my shower drain and sink, a remedy that is environmentally friendly. This might sound stupid in the context of this book, but nobody likes unclogging a drainpipe, certainly not when you have just massaged a hair mask into your hair.

DELICIOUSLY SMELLING OIL FOR EVERYDAY USE

My recipe with oils and essential oils for a fresh scent and light haircare. Take a little bottle with a drip counter of about 50 ml (1.7 fluid ounces) and mix 40 ml (1.35 fluid ounces) of oil like jojoba oil, argan oil or a mixture of your favourite oils.

Continue to fill the bottle with essential oils such as rose oil or lavender, ylang-ylang or a mix of your own choice. Shake the bottle well before each use, apply a few drops to the palm of your hand and then gently rub your hands together. Massage the oil into the lengths of your hair to take care of the ends and to soften frizzy hair and make it smooth. Caution: a little goes a long way and 'less is more' when using oils.

I love to use the essential oils from Young Living. They offer wonderful single and mixed formula's that meet the highest standards.
www.youngliving.com

ANTI-DANDRUFF OIL

You can make a natural anti-dandruff treatment yourself using tea tree essential oil.

Mix 100 ml (3.38 fluid ounces) of basic oil (e.g. olive oil, jojoba oil, almond oil...) with 20 drops of tea tree oil and 20 drops of eucalyptus oil. Shake the bottle thoroughly. Apply some oil to your hands, rub it between your hands and massage into your scalp. Let it sit for at least half an hour.

Especially the tea tree oil has a very strong scent, a bit like turpentine, but it really is worth using it. It is a bonus that it also wards off viruses during the cold season.

APPLE VINEGAR RINSE

To make your hair extra shiny and to rid your hair every now and then of residues from hair products, you can use apple vinegar. It's a grandmother's remedy that gives really good results. Apple vinegar makes sure that the hair sheaths close nicely, which makes your hair look smoother and shinier.

To do an apple vinegar rinse, take one part water and one part of organic apple vinegar (easily recognizable by the sediment at the bottom of the bottle and its turbid color). Use this rinse after your conditioner and let it work its magic for about a minute. Afterwards you can rinse your hair with fresh water.

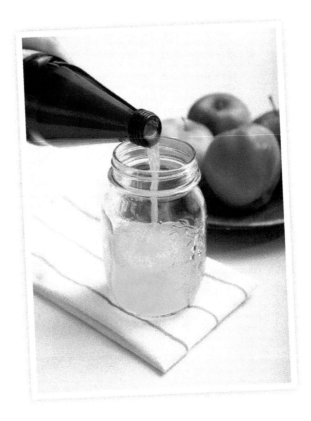

ANTI-LICE REMEDY

It's annoying to see a school note in the backpack of your daughter or son that a lice infestation is 'back in school'. Not the most fun subject in this book, but as a mother I couldn't deny you this tip. To treat lice you can buy a remedy at your pharmacist's or supermarket, but you can also treat it the natural way with a home-made remedy. Besides the classical treatment using shampoo, conditioner and especially the combing with a fine-toothed lice comb, you can protect your little sweetheart by putting two drops of essential lavender oil on the crown of the head or under the ponytail each morning before going to school.

The scent smells deliciously relaxing for us but lice absolutely hate it.

Another good remedy is using an apple vinegar rinse. You can use the above recipe for that.

ACKNOWLEDGMENTS

This book would never have been created without the influence and support of many special people in my life.

To Gina, my wonderful daughter. You are the most beautiful birthday present I ever received. I hope that my projects, my passion and persistance inspire you to go for your dreams!

To mom and dad: from early childhood you have given me a deep feeling of love and respect for nature. These are values that have become an intrinsic part of my life and that I integrate fully into my many projects and companies. You have always supported me in all my endeavours, not always knowing what I was doing. Thank you for the special mark your education printed on the way I live my life.

To Kaat and Freek, my sister and brother: we are all passionate creatures. Three totally different individuals who support eachother through thick and thin each from our own expertise. I love you!

Serge: life gave us something beautiful: our gorgeous daughter Gina. From a difficult period in our marriage we were able to build a new form of a family and a relationship based on love, respect and friendship. Thank you for everything.

It takes a village… to combine a busy life with the caretaking of my fantastic daughter. Thank you to everyone that is a part of my special family:
Odette, for your unconditional and warm love
Tine, you have the greatest heart of all, I am glad you came into our family
Caroline and Carlos, for your support, friendship and taxi-services;))
Nordine, Louisa, Lina, Lilia, Rebecca, Finn, Marit
Pieter-Jan, Monica and kids: thank you for your friendship
Vanessa, for your neverending love for our Gina

Ben Verleysen, Jürgen Sinnaeve, Any Uyttersprot, Rudy Galle and Johan Van Waeyenberge: all the people that have supported my projects from the early beginning with their expertise and their network. Thank you for sharing the belief in my dreams.

Paul and Cathérine De Poot, for the pleasant cooperation and the trust in our partnership.
Bernard Kint, dermatologist, for proofreading the scientific information.
Christine Verstraete, Gom-Magie "Specialist in wood renovation": thank you for using your cosy house as the setting for the photoshoots and for being a great neighbour!
Alain Verlinde, Eyeobject for the professional help making the promotional video's for this book.
My gratitude to Kristof Lamberigts and especially to your highly professional and enthousiastic team: Anne-Sophie Moerman, Cleo Vandenbosch, Kim Van Kerckhoven, Joni Verhulst, Wendy De Vlaeminck and all people behind the scenes. To Dirk Alexander for the beautiful photographs in this book and the pleasant photoshoot.

To my dear friends Saskia Winkler, Sally Gray and Haylie Pomroy: because of your input this book is filled with experiences from your practices. Your expertise and knowledge is priceless. I am eternally grateful for this and so happy that you crossed my life path.
To Tanja: without your "kutchi kutchi" life would be soooo boring!

Jack Canfield and his amazing team: thank you for your transformational words and thank you for showing me the way to get to where I want to be.

To all people involved in the creation and production of Delphin & Emerence. Your craftsmanship and the love for your profession are incredible.
To the team from Ark Communication: I hope that one day I will have a team as fun and competent as yours!

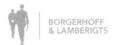
BORGERHOFF
& LAMBERIGTS

GHENT, BELGIUM
INFO@BORGERHOFF-LAMBERIGTS.BE
WWW.BORGERHOFF-LAMBERIGTS.BE

GHENT, BELGIUM
INFO@BORGERHOFF-LAMBERIGTS.BE
WWW.BORGERHOFF-LAMBERIGTS.BE

ISBN 9789089317506
Nur 453
D2017/11.089/16

AUTHOR Lies Helsloot
PHOTOGRAPHY Dirk Alexander, Istock
REVISION Katarina D'Hooge
COORDINATION Anne-Sophie Moerman, Cleo Vandenbosch & Joni Verhulst
DESIGN & TYPESETTING Wendy De Vlaeminck

Original version: 'Het complete boek over haar'
ISBN: 9789089317018
First print 2017

Many thanks to Charlotte Doolaege, Haylie Pomroy, Saskia Winkler, Sally Gray

MEER INFORMATIE
WWW.TAKEYOUTIME.COM
Sally Gray ND: www.sallygraynd.com
Saskia Winkler, coach and mentor: www.saskia-winkler.com
Haylie Pomroy, nutritionist: www.hayliepomroy.com
Jack Canfield, life coach and author: www.jackcanfield.com

DISCLAIMER